INTRODUC
TO THE
TECHNIQ

PRAISE FOR
INTRODUCTION TO THE ALEXANDER TECHNIQUE

"

I came to the Alexander Technique rather late in my career and have found it to be incredibly useful as an actress and singer. Bill Connington is an outstanding teacher, and if you can't study personally with him, this book is the next best thing! The Alexander Technique has helped me deal with the anxiety I sometimes feel, and I have become much freer on stage. The exercises in this book are a regular part of my preparation for any kind of performance. I wish I had discovered it sooner.

LIZ CALLAWAY
Broadway and recording star
Emmy Award winner; Tony Award nominee

"

Often acting is described by its gurus in ethereal and mystical terms, leaving performers scratching their heads as to how to unscramble the puzzle. The Alexander Technique thus becomes a rubric, allowing students to begin the process of deciphering this riddle by providing a practical and chiefly physical exploration of the self. In this book, Bill Connington further distills the technique to give students a lifetime of tools for the mining of the self, a necessity for any would-be performer dreaming of the grandiose.

JULIAN ELIJAH MARTINEZ
Broadway and television actor
MFA, Yale School of Drama

"

With the same gentle ease he brings to the classroom, Bill Connington offers encouraging prose that provides clarity to essential elements of the actor's practice and takes us step-by-step toward a more integrated self—one in which mind and body are connected and, with the release of unnecessary tension, one in which our creative impulses are free to flow. The simplicity with which he makes profound concepts accessible and inspires each of us to bring awareness to our breath and bodies through easy-to-follow exercises is extraordinary. *Introduction to the Alexander Technique* gives student actors an essential grounding in the principles of the technique and a foundation from which they may use their voices and bodies to express the truth of any character.

EVAN YIONOULIS
Richard Rodgers Director of Drama, the Juilliard School
Obie Award–winning director

In *Introduction to the Alexander Technique*, my colleague Bill Connington captures the essence of the Alexander Technique as it relates to actor training. With clarity and dynamic style, he inspires greater awareness of the body-mind connection and provides actors with strategies to release tension, a primary challenge for performing artists. Actors will refer to Bill's guidance again and again as they develop balance, ease, and awareness in their work. Contained in these pages are the secrets of a lifelong discipline.

JESSICA WOLF
Professor in the Practice of Acting, Yale School of Drama

A distillation of Bill Connington's many years of work as both an actor and teacher of the Alexander Technique, *Introduction to the Alexander Technique* provides student actors with many clear and practical ways of working on themselves. The tone is calm and supportive, nonjudgmental and encouraging. Bill makes the process utterly accessible while honoring the multiple elements required to develop one's instrument for the profession. He speaks with deep psychophysical understanding. I find the book a gift, a reference that the actor will be able to return to and draw from over and over again.

KIM JESSOR
Alexander faculty, Graduate Acting Program and New Studio on Broadway, NYU Tisch School of the Arts

As a speaker, I've found Connington's work with the Alexander Technique to be a huge asset. Reading *Introduction to the Alexander Technique* provides truly impressive relief from the stress and tension that stop performers from giving all they have inside them. The clarity with which Bill explains how to melt away stress and restore the full freedom needed by actors, musicians, and speakers—anyone who wants to connect to an audience—is nothing less than a small miracle. You'll find yourself reading the book over and over.

BARBARA SHER
New York Times bestselling author of I Could Do Anything If I Only Knew What It Was: How to Discover What You Really Want and How to Get It

Introduction to the Alexander Technique is written with an eloquent precision that guides readers effortlessly through an active physical and mental expansion. The practical exercises are a goldmine! Readers can fully embody their potential by learning to center themselves, energize, deepen their presence, and even send text messages with more radiance and flow.

JANE GUYER FUJITA
Assistant Arts Professor, Graduate Acting Program,
NYU Tisch School of the Arts

Bill Connington has written a book that not only explains the Alexander Technique in clear, simple, and accessible language but also reveals to the young actor the technique's value for the art of acting. Bill's empathetic and supportive voice and the exercises he includes immediately awaken the student's self-awareness and mind–body connection; reading it is a rich experiential journey.

CAROLYN SEROTA
Alexander faculty, Drama Division, the Juilliard School

The Alexander Technique should be an essential part of every young actor's training, and this book lays the foundation for that process. Balancing theory with real-world applications and practical exercises, Bill Connington brings the Alexander Technique on par with the movement, voice, and acting segments of the typical curriculum and has created a valuable resource for drama students and Alexander Technique teachers alike. I look forward to using *Introduction to the Alexander Technique* with my students!

LISA LEVINSON
Chair, American Society for the Alexander Technique
Adjunct Faculty, Carnegie Mellon School of Drama

For the undergraduate actor, self-awareness is vital to the development of artistic gifts. In *Introduction to the Alexander Technique*, Bill Connington gives the actor useful and creative exercises that tease out the principles of the technique in ways that are practical, accessible, and fun.

GEORDIE MACMINN
Professor, School of Drama,
University of North Carolina School of the Arts

INTRODUCTION TO THE ALEXANDER TECHNIQUE

A Practical Guide for Actors

Bill Connington

methuen | drama

LONDON • NEW YORK • OXFORD • NEW DELHI • SYDNEY

METHUEN DRAMA
Bloomsbury Publishing Plc
50 Bedford Square, London, WC1B 3DP, UK
1385 Broadway, New York, NY 10018, USA

BLOOMSBURY, METHUEN DRAMA and the Methuen Drama logo are trademarks of
Bloomsbury Publishing Plc

First published in Great Britain 2020

Series design by Charlotte Daniels
Cover image © Troyek / Getty Images

A catalogue record for this book is available from the British Library.

A catalog record for this book is available from the Library of Congress.

ISBN: HB: 978-1-3500-5294-9
           PB: 978-1-3500-5295-6
           ePDF: 978-1-3500-5293-2
           eBook: 978-1-3500-5296-3

Series: Acting Essentials

Typeset by Integra Software Services Pvt. Ltd.
Printed and bound in India

To find out more about our authors and books visit www.bloomsbury.com
and sign up for our newsletters.

For the faculty, staff, and students of the
Yale School of Drama—my inspiring
and inspired colleagues

CONTENTS

FOREWORD: TO THE YOUNG WHO WANT TO

The book you are holding in your hands may well become one of the most valuable resources in your personal library—one of those works one feels compelled to return to again and again for inspiration, guidance, solace, and sound practical advice. This book deserves your attention: within these pages are words and phrases that need to be highlighted, paragraphs that need to be underlined, and margins that should be written into. This is a book you can invest in.

The Alexander Technique occupies a central place in the curriculum of some of the best-known actor training programs in North America and Europe, including the Yale School of Drama, where I teach alongside my colleague Bill Connington, the author of this book. Bill has done a masterly job of introducing the fundamental principles of the technique and has provided a progression of basic exercises that gives you, dear reader, the opportunity to directly apply those principles both in your ordinary daily routine and in your work as a performing artist—in class, in rehearsal, and on stage in front of an audience. Consider this an owner's manual, a workbook for your mind, body, and spirit, an introduction to a practice that can help you access your creative instincts and emotional life and humanity with awareness, presence, and a kind of relaxed availability, all of which will make you a better actor.

The Alexander Technique requires dealing with cause rather than effect. The exercises Bill describes in this book are concerned with rethinking the way you use yourself rather than with "fixing" your alignment or "correcting" the way you move. You must sacrifice your desire for results to the experience of cause. To work on your body—and by extension, on your breath, your voice, and your acting—relies as much on awareness and attention as it does on physical effort. If you try to engage in any activity through physical effort alone you will end up using more muscular force than is required, and there's a very good likelihood that you won't use the best muscles for the job. Employing mental focus and direction to stimulate activity leads to much more accurate and efficient use of the muscles, which means that these activities are carried out with greater ease and flexibility. This is the kind of technique that interests me: one that can help you do your best work and help you feel free and creative wherever and with whomever you are working.

This can become a *daily* practice. If you earnestly engage yourself in the study of the Alexander Technique, there is no end to where this work can lead you. The simplicity and subtlety of Alexander's work is astonishing. Once you finish going through this book for the first time, cycle back to the first chapter and mindfully practice the entire sequence of exercises again. Doing something again and again and again is the only way for actors to let go of psychophysical habits that do not serve them, enabling them to build a new and more useful way of working. Repetition builds strength and confidence. Every time you return to the beginning, it may feel like a different experience because you will have changed, and your relationship to yourself and to your body will have changed—and that's one way you know you're making progress.

As someone who is committed to raising the standard of practice in the field, I'm grateful to Bill for sharing his expertise so generously and with his customary grace and clarity. If you are intent on improving your craft and becoming a more versatile and accomplished storyteller, I encourage you to take advantage of what this book offers and get down to work.

Walton Wilson
Chair, Department of Acting
Yale School of Drama
May 2019

SERIES INTRODUCTION

Acting Essentials is the first book series specifically intended for undergraduate students of drama. The books in the series are not theoretical; rather, they are practical. Fifty percent of the text consists of exercises designed to help the reader learn the material and apply it directly to rehearsals, auditions, and performances.

The series is comprehensive and aims to cover everything the undergraduate needs to know about performance. Classical and contemporary acting, acting for the camera, voice, speech, the business of acting, musical theater, and the Alexander Technique are all foundational topics for any acting program.

The books are also designed to speak to a large and diverse group of students. Diversity and inclusion are necessary because our world is diverse. Drama students come from all kinds of backgrounds and points of view, and so do the Acting Essentials authors. Moreover, the series is designed to remove geographic barriers to top-level instruction in drama. In the past, students often needed to study in New York, Los Angeles, or London to be able to work with well-known experts in the field. Acting Essentials makes the knowledge of those experts available to all students, regardless of where they study.

The Acting Essentials authors are highly experienced and respected. They are teachers and chairs of departments, but they are also practitioners—actors, directors, and writers. They speak their truths from a deep and deeply known place. Their voices are friendly, supportive, constructive, and enlightening. In essence, they have written workbooks that will show you the nuts and bolts of the acting craft. When craft is mastered, art can bloom.

To begin the study of acting is exciting and sometimes daunting. There is so much to learn—where to begin? The authors of Acting Essentials speak with authoritative guidance, ready to pass their knowledge to succeeding generations. While building on the great traditions of the past, they are firmly rooted in contemporary artistry.

Studying acting is a journey, both into a new field of endeavor and into the self. This two-pronged journey is both outwardly and inwardly directed. Acting Essentials will lay the foundation for this lifelong journey, from the first flicker of intention all the way through the challenges of the professional world.

To quote the great Nigerian novelist Chinua Achebe, "There is no story that is not true." The Acting Essentials series is here to help every actor tell truthful stories.

Bill Connington
Lecturer in Acting, Yale School of Drama
New York and New Haven
April 2019

ACKNOWLEDGMENTS

Many thanks to friends and colleagues for their help with this project:

To everyone at Methuen Drama: Meredith Benson, Lucy Brown, Camilla Erskine, John O'Donovan, Jenny Ridout, and especially Anna Brewer for seeing the book through to publication.

To my literary agent, Barbara Clark.

To my Yale School of Drama colleagues Jessica Wolf and Walton Wilson for reviewing the manuscript and to the institution itself for giving me an artistic home.

To those who read parts of the book in manuscript form: Melissa Glueck, Jenny Cline, Laura Parker, Deirdre Broderick, Doireann Mac Mahon, and John Evans Reese.

To Michael Cooper, Deirdre Broderick, and Lauren Schiff for their friendship and support.

To Rebecca Margolick for her invaluable work assisting me in the preparation of the manuscript.

To my musical colleague David Sytkowski for his insight and sensitivity in team teaching.

To Sophie Gillespie for copyediting the text and project manager Damian Penfold for overseeing the publication process.

And to my friend and colleague Barbara Sher for her inspiration and example.

ABOUT THE EXERCISES

One of the most important things about the Alexander Technique is its usefulness. Theory is unhelpful unless there is a clear and direct pragmatic application. This book and these exercises are all about supporting you in your acting work and the mind–body aspect of daily life.

You will find the exercises grouped together at the end of each chapter. I call them core exercises because they summarize the most important aspects of the text that precedes them. In addition, each chapter contains what I call a primary exercise, one that encapsulates all the chapter's important concepts in one activity.

Work through the whole book, then find the exercises that are most helpful to you. Make a list, then practice ten minutes a day, whenever you can fit it into your schedule. In this way, the Alexander principles become an organic part of your life. Unlike yoga and meditation, the Alexander Technique doesn't require you to set aside twenty, thirty, or even sixty minutes a day for practice. Ten minutes is enough—or you can practice twice a day for five minutes each. Even practicing for two to three minutes, if you do it each day, will heighten your sensory awareness, help you recognize your habits, and ease you into new ways of being.

You don't need any special equipment to do the exercises, but you may wish to have a few ordinary objects at hand—a slim paperback book to put under your head when you're lying on the floor; a folding chair; a blank book or journal in which you can record your thoughts. Your smartphone may even play a role in some of the exercises.

Video versions of these exercises are available free of charge at https://vimeo.com/channels/1488540. A complete library of Alexander Technique exercises that I specifically devised for students is also available, at https://vimeo.com/channels/connington. The videos will help you understand my practical and exploratory approach to the Alexander Technique; they're not meant to be followed as a strict protocol. The goal is to help you use yourself with increased freedom and ease, resulting in a more creative, bolder artist: you.

INTRODUCTION

Empathy is at the heart of the actor's art.

**MERYL STREEP, COMMENCEMENT SPEECH AT
BARNARD COLLEGE, MAY 2010**

You are studying acting. Something about the alchemy of theater and film drew you in. What attracted you to theatrical storytelling? Perhaps you acted as a child or in high school. Or maybe it was the allure of "becoming someone else," the excitement of collaborating with other creative people, the fun of rehearsing and working toward a collective goal: the performance. And possibly the most powerful draw of all was the experience—even if you had it only once or twice—of knowing that the audience was leaning forward to *hear* you and really *see* you. It's like nothing else.

And yet sometimes something gets in the way. It's hard to pin down. Some acting classes go better than others. Some rehearsals go well, others less so. Sometimes you land a role in the play, sometimes you don't. Of course you can't control when you get cast, but you can strive to always do your best work.

These are issues that almost every actor has to grapple with. *How* does one always do one's best in class, rehearsal, audition, and performance? What is the key to staying connected to the truth of the character and the scene? What is the first step to *unlocking and unblocking* your natural talent so it flows naturally?

If I had to choose two things that I see stop performers most often, they would be excessive tension and negative self-judgment. These two often appear in tandem.

Every actor has experienced fear, stress, and anxiety at some point. It's true: performance situations are always more heightened than everyday life, and it feels like there is a lot at stake. A state of excitement mixed with a bit of nervousness will probably always be there when you perform, but there is a point where nerves and tension get in the way. Teachers often exhort students to use their nerves in performance, but they don't tell them *how* to do so. Nerves get in the way of artistic impulses, creativity, and spontaneity. It's almost as if worry and anxiety clog up the actor's instrument, which is the *self*. What can you do to unblock it?

DEFINING THE ALEXANDER TECHNIQUE

The Alexander Technique is a method of education through which you learn how to recognize your unconstructive mind–body habits, consciously prevent them, and develop more positive and efficient ways of functioning by mentally cuing yourself.

Many college and university drama departments and performing arts conservatories turn to the Alexander Technique[1] as a vital part of a performer's training. The technique is named after F. Matthias Alexander (1869–1955), an Australian actor and teacher. When Alexander was a young man, he was a one-man reciter of Shakespeare, which was a common form of entertainment before radio, TV, and film became popular. Alexander's difficulty was that he suffered from chronic hoarseness when performing, sometimes even losing his voice.

When doctors and voice teachers were unable to help, Alexander set out to solve the problem himself. At the time, he was working as an actor with his own theater company and running one of the world's first drama schools. He decided to observe his own movement and functioning closely, both in daily life and when he practiced his orations at home, in front of a three-way mirror. He discovered that his head–neck relationship was unbalanced. When he started to speak, his neck would

---

[1]In addition to your work in school, I would recommend that you take lessons with a certified Alexander Technique teacher to facilitate your learning process. The method can be learned in small group classes or in private one-on-one lessons. The teacher uses verbal instruction and gentle hands-on guidance to help students find new and constructive ways to reduce tension.

tighten and his head would pull back and down toward his shoulders, which caused a chain reaction of downward pressure through his torso and the rest of his body.

This series of tensions caused tightness and stiffness in his throat and indirectly caused his vocal difficulties. Over time he was able to stop himself before he tightened up. This pause would leave his neck gently elongated, his head balanced at the top of his spine, and his torso naturally at its full height. Indirectly this took care of his hoarseness, and he stopped losing his voice. *When Alexander stopped interfering with his natural mind–body coordination (i.e., when he stopped tensing up), his use of himself—his functioning—improved markedly.*

After solving his own difficulties, Alexander then devoted the rest of his long life to teaching his mind–body method to others. He worked in London and New York with well-known actors and people in the fields of science, education, and government. He was at the vanguard of what we would now call *somatic education*. The legacy of F. M. Alexander continues to influence thousands of people working in the theater and film worlds. His work is like a pebble dropped in water, with ever-expanding outward concentric circles. His influence will continue to be deeply influential for the foreseeable future.

The Alexander Technique is ultimately very practical. It helps you catch yourself when you are slumping over as you learn lines or sit at the computer. It calls your attention to situations where your alignment is off or your movement is jerky or tight. It helps you become aware of when you are holding your breath, pushing your voice, or not listening to your scene partner. It is one of the most pragmatic ways actors can help themselves.

This book will show you many ways that you can help yourself through the Alexander Technique, whether in class, rehearsal, audition, or performance. It will help you find the subtle balance and coordination that integrates all aspects of yourself: mind, body, emotions, breath, voice, and creative impulses. In essence, the technique can help you be more fully yourself.

But don't you want to be someone else when you're acting? Partly. Because even if you are pulling off a major transformation and playing a character who is nothing like yourself, you are still "using yourself" in order to bring that character to life. It's your voice, your emotions, your body that help create that character on the stage or film set. And you want to fine-tune the instrument that is yourself so that you can give the best performance possible.

One of the most important things you can learn in drama training is how to focus on the *process* of acting rather than the *results*. Giving your attention to the *how* of acting will indirectly affect the end result. Rather than attempting to be a "good actor giving a good performance," you attempt to play your character in the character's given circumstances. This may sound obvious, but it's easy to get off track when you are trying to do a lot of things at once.

The Alexander Technique will help you get on track and stay on it by reducing tension, freeing up your breathing, and releasing your body. Releasing your body will in turn help you release your mind, unlock your emotions, increase your spontaneity, and reinforce your creative impulses. The Alexander Technique does this by showing you that you have many more choices than you realize, in your acting and your life. And choices are the doorway to freedom: to act, to perform, to do whatever you want to do.

You can work through this book methodically in eight weeks, as it is laid out on the page. Read one chapter a week, do a few exercises per day, and at the end of the eight weeks, you'll feel like a different actor and a different person—or, rather, you will feel more like yourself than you did before. Or you can simply dip into the book wherever you like. Do whatever exercises you want, in whatever order you want. Either way, you will begin to realize how you might change yourself profoundly by being more profoundly yourself. After all, that's what the audience wants to see—your most essential, unadorned self in performance. We're all looking forward to seeing that. So let's get started.

1 YOUR BODY

The beginning is the most important part of the work.
                                        PLATO, *REPUBLIC*, BOOK II

In the beginning, there was your body. As a newly born child, you were all body, movement, and emotion. Formulated thoughts came later. Newborns and young children move naturally and freely as an expression of who they are and what they want. For the actor, it is the same: *motivation leads to action.* Your physicality and movement are an expression of who you are and what you want as the character you are playing. Fortunately, you already have experience connecting with your body in this way from early childhood.

A bit later in life, maybe after the age of seven or eight, many of us begin to develop tension habits. Those habits can interfere with movement, functioning, alignment, and even the mind–body connection. But I'm getting a little ahead of myself. I'll come back to this in a bit.

If you're reading this book sequentially, this is another kind of beginning: the first week of an eight-week program. We'll consider a different aspect of your self each week.

If you're skipping around the book nonsequentially: great. You'll be reading about various parts of yourself, but in a different order. However you go through this process, at the end you'll be putting all the components together to form a whole: *an integrated you.*

For the actor, as for any performing artist, your body is like a canvas on which you paint—a physical manifestation of an inner state of mind that makes creative expression possible. Without your body, you cannot act.

But *what is your body?* Of course it's a number of parts: your torso, arms, legs, head, hands, and feet. But how are the parts integrated? How does it all work together in a harmonious whole to create the performance you want?

Many actors have no idea. Answer the three questions in the box below as a first step toward finding out. Write your answers on a piece of paper, or in your phone. There are no right answers—just the answers that are right for you.

QUESTIONS FOR YOUR INNER SELF

1 What are you aware of right now in your own body?
2 What do you think a "good actor's body" is?
3 What is the central coordinating system for your body and your movement?

Sensory Awareness and a "Good Actor's Body"

To answer the first question, you must make use of your **sensory awareness**. We all understand the physical senses of sight, hearing, smell, taste, and touch. Sensory awareness is a bit different. It gives you a sense of your inner and outer environment. It helps create your understanding of your body in space, its positioning and movement, and how much effort it takes to create that movement. As you train as an actor, you'll find that sensory awareness will become one of your most valuable tools.

The more you use your sensory awareness effectively, the more accurate it becomes. If you're not used to using a sense, it gets a little rusty. For example, if you're not used to looking closely at things, you might have a little trouble distinguishing between subtle shades of green and blue. But the more you're aware of your visual sense, the easier it is to discern differences. It's the same with sensory awareness. The more you use it, the more accurately you'll be able to track where your body is in space and what it's doing.

You will have your own answer to the second question. Of course it's always desirable for the actor to have a strong, flexible body. But a "good actor's body" doesn't necessarily have to mean muscular. And by "good body," I don't mean a specific body type. There are so many types of characters to play. My personal definition of a "good actor's body" is one that is well integrated, balanced, flexible, and ready to act. You might consider this a new definition of what a good actor's body is. This book will show you how to develop that.

The Central Coordinating System

In the Alexander Technique, the key to central coordination is called the **head-neck relationship**—i.e., the way your head is balanced at the top of your spine. When it's well balanced, it helps organically coordinate your whole body. When your neck is free and released, your head can be poised and balanced. This helps everything below it—torso, arms, hands, legs, and feet—work more gracefully and efficiently as well as in unison. This is called constructive coordination.

But what does this all have to do with acting? Well: everything. The way you walk, run, sit, stand, bend, talk, and breathe is affected by your sensory awareness and your head-neck relationship. If you are tight, tense, or stiff, this will decrease your ability to access an accurate sensory awareness, and it will tend to tighten your neck and contract your head down onto your spine. This in turn puts downward pressure on your whole body, so it gets tight. Alignment is thrown off, and all your movements are affected—often getting heavier, jerkier, and less efficient.

To make things a bit more complex, if you're used to being tight, tense, and stiff, then it *becomes harder to feel.* Tension starts to feel normal. But other people can see it. Your acting, singing, and movement teachers are trained to discern tension and other physical issues in their students, and sometimes they may mention it to you. It's always easier to see habits in someone else. You, too, may notice physical mannerisms in your friends, classmates, or people on the street. Once you pay attention to it, it's easy to spot people who have:

- slumping posture,
- a neck that juts forward,
- arching in the lower back,
- raised shoulders,
- a body that pulls to one side or the other, or
- a head that retracts back.

Tension Habits

But don't worry: *if your body has learned to be tight, it can also learn to release*. The main objective is to target your **tension habits**. We all have them. Even the simplest physical activities—sitting at the computer, reaching for a cup of coffee, driving a car—can have strong habits associated with them. In fact, the simplest movements and activities often go along with the strongest tension habits. Tension gets ingrained in these habitual movements because we "don't need to think about them." In some way the body comes to feel that it *needs* to tense in order to carry out a movement. Of course this is not true. Your body may overwork itself when it's trying to help you carry out various simple activities.

QUESTIONS FOR YOUR INNER SELF

1 How do you define tension?
2 What are your personal manifestations of tension?
3 How might it be possible to change your tension habits?

I bring this up because *tension may be the actor's number one problem*. It may stop your creative flow, get you locked in your head, and even contribute to performance anxiety. But when you effectively address tension and its domino-like side effects, you are well on your way to being "in the zone."

You can define "tension" in many different ways. My definition is simple and easy to remember. Every action in the body takes a certain amount of muscular effort. Any effort that is more than necessary I would define as tension. For example, to lift your arm takes the coordinated action of muscles in your arm and supporting muscles in your shoulder and back. But if, like many people, you stiffen your neck, tighten and lift your shoulder, and maybe even squeeze your breath a bit as you lift your arm, I would call that tension.

There is a nearly infinite variety of possible physical habits born of tension. Some people slump down when they raise their arms. Some stiffen the back and lift the shoulders. Others do a combination of both. As you begin to become conscious of your movement using your sensory awareness, you'll notice all kinds of patterns—some subtle, others less so. There will be much more about this in the movement chapter.

Allowing for Change

How might it be possible to change? This all relates to your **mind**-**set**, which is essentially a series of ideas, concepts, and assumptions that influence the way you see yourself and the world. We all have a mind-set: there are as many of them as there are individuals. But some people think they *must* do this or that to change their way of viewing things.

My theory of change is different. *I believe it's not desirable to force change but rather to allow it.* If you try to force your body to do something, it may rebel. This goes for the mind and emotions, too.

In my view, the way to allow change to happen is to *set an intention and to stay with that intention gently yet persistently.*

Further, it will make your work much easier if you maintain a *constructive, growth-oriented mind-set.* It will open the door to all kinds of creative impulses and will let you approach each new acting challenge with openness and flexibility.

QUESTIONS FOR YOUR INNER SELF

1   How would you define positive change?
2   How do you start on and follow a path of constructive change?
3   Where does change lead you?

When I'm looking to make any kind of change in myself, I find it valuable to go through the following steps:

- Take stock of where I am at present.

- Get clear about what it is I'd like to change.

- Make a pragmatic plan for change that I can actually stick to.

- Touch base periodically to reassess.

Tough-love tactics and the "just do it" philosophy may be effective for some people. But in my teaching experience, I've seen that it's challenging for most students to be motivated by that philosophy and stick with it over the long term. If it works for you, great. But for the rest of us, a softer approach may be easier to follow. Part of that approach involves understanding why you've done things a certain way in the past. Then you can acknowledge that your circumstances have changed and make the decision to do things in a new way.

I prefer not to use "tough talk" to change my mind-set when I catch myself falling into old patterns. For example, I used to arch my back quite a bit in daily life. Even now, after studying and teaching Alexander Technique for many years, occasionally I catch myself arching my back if I'm tired or not feeling well. *It's normal to sometimes fall back into old habits and ways of being.* But when I become aware of an old pattern, I can do something about it.

I find it helpful to take an almost scientific approach, meaning self-talk along the lines of, "Oh, isn't that interesting? When I get tense, I hold my breath, stiffen my neck, and tense my shoulders." In other words, I attempt to *not blame myself*, and this helps me develop new and more constructive ways of doing things.

For me, developing a path of change also involves coming to a temporary halt. Sitting down and taking stock. Looking at the issues from all angles. Life is often a long to-do list, and we jump from one task to another. It's a luxury to take a meditative break to think things through. A focused five or ten minutes—or even two minutes—without looking at a phone or a computer and just *thinking* can really make a difference.

The question "Where does change lead you?" is really a **Socratic question**—i.e., one that stimulates you to come to your own conclusion and encourages you to examine your own thoughts and thinking processes. The question has no one correct answer. Some people might respond with "into the unknown," "to someplace new," or "to a different part of myself." Whatever your answer is, write it down and put it where you can refer to it periodically. And see if your answer evolves over time.

Definition of the Alexander Process

The Alexander Technique involves a unique *three-step process*:

1 Sensory awareness
2 Inhibition
3 Direction

We've already discussed the first step—sensory awareness. The next step is a brief stop, or pause. In that split second, we remind ourselves *consciously* that we don't want to maintain whatever old, inefficient habit we're trying to break.

In that moment, which I call *a moment of suspension*, you tell yourself, "I don't want to tighten. I don't want to hold on to my old habit." The moment of suspension is what F. M. Alexander called **inhibition**—i.e., inhibiting, or saying no, to an old habit.

WHAT IS INHIBITION?

After becoming aware of an unconstructive habit, you pause for a split second to remind yourself that you don't want to continue it. This is what is sometimes called a "positive no."

Inhibition is the step that it is easy to forget. You become aware of something in yourself you want to change—"My shoulders are rounded forward"; "My teacher told me my neck is jutting forward, which restricts my voice"—and consciously decide you don't want to do it anymore.

You have a split second between getting the idea to do something and carrying out the action. If you say no to your old habit in that split second, you leave yourself open to something new.

WHAT ARE MY ALEXANDER DIRECTIONS?

The term "direction" refers to a specific type of thinking, or mental cuing. This takes the form of gentle guidance:

- Let my neck be free
- To let my head release forward and up
- To let my torso lengthen and widen
- To let my arms and legs release away from my body

These classic Alexander Technique directions allow the body to "flow" up and out, naturally and organically. The more you practice these thoughts, the more easily your body will respond and retain them in a positive manner.

The third step in the process is called *directing*. In contemporary language we would call this *mental cuing*. It helps to think of directing as synonymous with *intention*. After all, intention is everything for the actor. "What is your objective?" is a classic question teachers ask students when they're working on a role. Your intention, or what you want, is also important for us in life.

Intention, Tension, and Context

There are three elements to intention:

- context,
- clarity, and
- follow-through.

Context is the big picture, such as the history and the world of the play or the background behind something you'd like to change in your daily life. Clarity is the specifics—the details of what you want to do. And following through means gently yet persistently reminding yourself of what you want, which is what you do when you think your Alexander Technique directions.

TENSION DOESN'T ELIMINATE TENSION

Often, when we try to "fix" a physical issue, it doesn't work. Why? Because fixing is results-oriented rather than process-oriented.

For example, if you pull yourself up straighter while sitting, standing, or walking, *you are using tension to attempt to fix a tension issue.* So your body can't maintain that position for longer than a couple of minutes. It's stiff, uncomfortable, and unsustainable.

What most people do when they attempt to improve their "bad posture" is pull themselves up from their backs. In so doing, the back stiffens, holds, and rigidifies. That in turn influences the shoulders and neck, encouraging them to tighten. Even the arms and legs get into the act.

Remember that when you're dealing with the body, which is what you use in acting, you cheat yourself if you try to *force* changes. You can go so much deeper if you *allow* them. Yes, we know that excessive tension is not good for us and that it restricts breathing, movement, and even how well we think. We also know that the body needs to be reminded of this. It needs to be reminded many times, because habits are so strong. But reminding is not the same as admonishing. Rather, it's gentle— the way you would talk to a good friend.

The Use of the Self and Alexander Directions

During the course of his work, F. M. Alexander coined the phrase "**the use of the self**," which means the way you function mentally, physically, and even emotionally in your daily life. For example, before an audition, you might become very nervous, not prepare anything until the night before (even though you had more time than that), and then, as you practice, tense your rib cage, hold your breath, tense your shoulders, tighten your neck, and pull your head back and down. A different use of the self might involve feeling a little nervous but also excited, spending as much time practicing as you can, and preparing physically through Alexander work and stretching.

To review, this is the Alexander process:

1 Sensory awareness

2 Inhibition

3 Direction

Initially you will need to think about and practice each of these components separately. But eventually the three components will become one organic whole. For example, you may catch yourself slumping. Catching yourself slumping is the first step (sensory awareness). Reminding yourself that you don't want to slump is the second step (inhibition). The third step is mentally cuing yourself with your Alexander directions. And your Alexander directions are:

- Let my neck be free
- To let my head release forward and up
- To let my torso lengthen and widen
- To let my arms and legs release away from my body

So rather than catching yourself slumping and pulling yourself up, you allow your body to transform organically and thus more effectively. As you gain experience practicing the Alexander Technique, you'll be able to improve the use of your self in activity as well. For example, you can become aware of yourself slumping as you're walking, and you'll be able to inhibit your old habits and direct yourself as you walk. Therefore, you'll be able to change your walk as you move.

Now it's time to put what we've learned in this chapter into practice.

JOURNAL

Find time to sit with your journal at some point this week. Your journal can be either on paper, on your computer, or on your phone. Write about the following questions:

1   How does tension sometimes get in your way?
2   How does the mind–body connection affect your acting and your daily life?
3   What might you do over the course of the coming week to help work on the use of your self?
4   When in your day can you put aside five minutes to practice the Alexander Technique?

Exercises Part 1

ALEXANDER DIRECTIONS

- Sit in a relatively straight-backed chair, with your back against the back of the chair, your feet on the floor, and your hands in your lap.
- Slump on purpose, to sense what that's like.
- Let go of the slump.
- Sit in an overly straight, military-style posture.
- Let go of that forced alignment.
- Think through your Alexander directions: *let your neck be free, let your head go forward and up, let your torso lengthen and widen, and let your arms and legs release away from your body.*

Neither slumping nor maintaining a military-style posture is an ideal way of sitting. Rather, *allow* yourself to be at your full height. *Let* your sitting be *active and engaged* in a gentle way. Your back muscles and your core support you in a healthful manner. Practice sitting this way for one to two minutes a few times a day. It will start to feel natural to you as you have more experience of it.

Let me clarify one important point: some people pull their necks forward in space, so the neck is too far forward. Ideally, in time, with Alexander work, the neck comes into a natural, easy alignment with the rest of the spine.

Similarly, most of us retract the head back and down sometimes. That means the head tips back and the chin raises. The weight of the head then compresses down onto the neck and the entire spine. So there is downward pressure on the whole body. One of the most important concepts in Alexander Technique is relieving that pressure. Allowing the head to rotate slightly forward—say, a quarter of an inch—and up toward the ceiling helps relieve tension and pressure through the rest of the body.

RELEASING YOUR NECK

In this exercise, I ask you to place your index fingers at your ear channel. That is the approximate level where your head sits on top of your spine. This is higher than many people realize. Having a physical reminder of that location helps you not collapse your neck. To see that location in visual form, go to www.visiblebody.com/. There you will see the atlas and the axis, the first two vertebrae of the spine, which allow for head and neck movement.

- Sit in a relatively straight-backed chair, with your back against the back of the chair, your feet on the floor, and your hands in your lap.
- Think through the Alexander directions.
- Place a finger in each ear to remind you where the top of the spine is.
- Bring your fingers down. Leave your neck free. Slowly turn your head from side to side, as if you're saying no.
- Allow your neck to be easy. Gently nod your head up and down several times, as if you're saying yes.
- Combine the two movements: nod up and down as you turn your head from side to side.
- Return to center. Think your Alexander directions again.

Sense whether your neck might feel a bit different at the end of the exercise from the way it felt at the beginning of the exercise. A soft, pliable neck is one of the primary objectives of Alexander work. It helps reduce tension through the face and head, the shoulders, and, indirectly, the rest of the body. A released neck helps breathing, speaking, singing, and may even help reduce stage fright. If you can let go of your neck, you can let go of the rest of your body. Ironically, the neck is often one of the tightest parts of the body. So it will take repetition to remind yourself to gradually change your neck-tightening habits.

HEAD POISE

- Sit in a relatively straight-backed chair, with your back against the back of the chair and your feet on the floor.
- Leave your hands released as you place them on your neck.
- Deliberately do the wrong thing: slump and retract your head back and down.
- Let go of the head retraction.
- Pull yourself up into military-style posture.
- Let go of the military-style posture.
- Think through your Alexander directions.
- Allow your head to be balanced and poised on top of your spine—that is, not too far forward or too far back.

This exercise is designed to help you find a new use of the self, one in which the neck is gently elongated and the head is balanced at the top of your spine. Your hands will help you feel what you're doing in your neck, both in slumping and military posture. You'll probably feel too much tension in both those states of being.

The head–neck relationship is one of the fundamentals of the Alexander Technique. When you free your neck, it allows your head to be poised, which takes pressure off your whole torso. When you let this happen, there is more space and freedom for your lungs and all your other internal organs.

It's a relief to let go of squeezing and physical constraint. When this happens, movement and functioning is easier. Anything you do in a scene is easier: listening, talking, communicating, following your character's objectives. At first it may feel a bit unfamiliar, or it may even feel "too fancy" or "arrogant" to stand at your full height. But just imagine your favorite classical actors or top-level athletes: there's a good chance they aren't shy about letting their bodies occupy as much space as they need.

LENGTHENING AND WIDENING YOUR TORSO

- Stand with your feet a bit apart and your arms hanging by your sides.
- Slump on purpose. Feel the heaviness in your body.
- Return to neutral.
- Think through your Alexander directions.
- Allow yourself to lengthen. The head leads upward, and the rest of the body follows.
- Let your breath flow easily as your body lengthens and widens.

Most people have a tendency to slump or collapse down on themselves. The neck muscles tighten, which contracts the head onto the neck, shoulders, and whole body. A shortening and narrowing of the body is the result. Often teachers advise actors to *"take up your full space."* This is both a physical and a mental suggestion. It means to stand tall, at your full height and width, but it also has the effect of giving you a sense of inner confidence and presence.

Some think that a slumped body is "natural." This is not the case. If you watch small children, you'll see that they move freely and easily, most often taking up their full space. Each of us has experienced this already. Slumping is a *habitual*, not *natural* action. See what it's like to fill yourself up to your fullest dimensions.

OPENING YOUR SHOULDERS PART 1

- Stand with your feet slightly apart and your arms hanging by your sides.
- Notice your shoulders. Are they slumped forward? Are they pressed back? Check in a mirror if you aren't sure.
- Check to see if one shoulder is higher than the other.
- Think through your Alexander directions.
- Think of opening across your shoulders and chest, but don't push your shoulders back.

- Float your arms straight out to the side. Think wide through the chest and shoulders.
- Float your arms back down. Repeat three times.

OPENING YOUR SHOULDERS PART 2

- Stand at your full height, with your feet slightly apart and your arms hanging by your sides.
- Think through your Alexander directions.
- Float your arms all the way up to the ceiling. Leave your body long and your shoulders down.
- Float your arms down to your sides. Repeat three times.
- Now imagine you are doing the backstroke. Bring one arm at time up, back, and around behind you.

Repeat several times, allowing for a full range of motion through your shoulders and arms.

The shoulders allow some of the potentially freest movements of all the joints. However, it's very common for performers to round their shoulders forward and/or raise their shoulders toward their ears. Others unconsciously squeeze their arms into their sides, restricting breathing and the movement of their shoulders and arms.

Tense shoulders can be distracting for the audience to look at. A performer with tight shoulders can come off as somewhat held back, or even defensive. A free shoulder girdle gives the impression of openness and a positive vulnerability. Letting go of shoulder tension can make a striking difference in the impression an actor makes.

RELEASING YOUR ARMS

- Stand at your full height, with your feet slightly apart and your arms hanging by your sides.
- Think through your Alexander directions.

- Maintaining your full height, place each hand on the opposite shoulder.
- Gently hug yourself without raising or rounding your shoulders. Let your arms drape as you do this for thirty to forty-five seconds.
- Float your arms directly in front of you at shoulder level. Repeat three times.
- Float your arms up to the ceiling. First, release your wrists. Second, release your elbows. Third, let the weight of your arms drop them down by your sides. Repeat three times.

SOFTENING THROUGH YOUR HANDS

- Sit in a relatively straight-backed chair, with your back against the back of the chair and your feet on the floor.
- Place your hands easily in your lap, palms resting on your thighs.
- Remaining tall, look down at your hands, remembering the pivot point at the level of the ears.
- Have the intention to release your finger joints and palms.
- Pick up your right hand with your left. One at a time, take hold of each of your fingers and gently elongate it to help it lengthen.
- Repeat with your left hand picking up your right.

This is a way to free your hands without cracking your knuckles, which is not good for them.

We use our arms and hands all day long: getting dressed, eating, working at the computer, driving. With all that work, sometimes the muscles can become cramped, and the joints can become constricted. Sometimes we use too much force with our hands, and they became tight and "graspy." Often young actors say "I don't know what to do with my hands" when working on a scene. When you release tension from your arms and hands, you will use them more naturally when you're in character.

LETTING GO OF YOUR LEGS

- Sit on the edge of a chair with your feet on the floor.
- Think through your Alexander directions.
- Sense your "sitting bones" against the chair.
- Place your fingers at your hip sockets, at the fold where your legs meet your torso.
- Slowly and easily bring your knees together and apart, leaving your feet against the floor. Do this several times.
- Place your hands on top of your thighs. Think of your body lengthening up as your legs release away from your body. *It's an intention rather than an action.*
- Think of being released, or "easy," in your hips, knees, and ankles.
- See if you can move your foot a few inches to the left and right without overtightening your thigh muscles.

Even in a simple activity such as standing or siting, the way you use your legs is vital. So often the knees get locked, but the ankle and hip joints can also be compromised, which restricts movement. In sitting the legs can do much less. They don't need to work hard, yet many people find it challenging to let go of their legs when sitting in a chair or on the floor. Raising your awareness and practicing this exercise will help.

FREEING THE FEET

- Sit in a relatively straight-backed chair, with your back against the back of the chair and your bare feet on the floor.
- Remaining at your full height, look down at your feet.
- See if you can lift your toes off the floor without tensing your legs, ankles, or feet.

- Leaving yourself at your full height and your leg free, pick your foot up off the ground a few inches without tensing. Repeat with the other foot. Make sure you keep breathing easily.
- Point and flex your foot several times. Repeat with the other foot.

We use our feet all day long but tend to forget about them. The more our feet can lengthen and widen, the more the rest of the body can let go. When we are able to be soft and flexible in our feet, we can sense our connection to the ground and the rest of the body can feel supported.

CONSTRUCTIVE REST

- Lie down on the floor, on your back. Make sure you are lying on an exercise mat, rug, or carpet.
- Place a softcover book or two under your head so that it's raised two to three inches off the floor.
- Bend your knees and place your feet on the floor.
- Put your hands on your lower rib cage.
- Think through your Alexander directions as you lie there for five to ten minutes.
- When you're finished, gently roll onto one side. Place one of your hands on the floor and press down to bring yourself to a sitting position.

Each element of this exercise has a purpose. The paperback books help keep your head from collapsing back and down onto your neck. The bending of the knees helps your lower back release toward the floor. Placing your hands on your rib cage helps keep your shoulders open and allows you to sense your own breathing. While lying down you are supported by the floor, which helps you inhibit your old, unconstructive habits. Rolling onto your side rather than doing a sit-up will help you maintain your length as you come up off the floor.

Constructive rest is one of the most luxurious gifts you can give yourself. Make it part of your daily routine, like brushing your teeth. It's a positive and constructive habit. By allowing your mind and body to take a break from constant activity, you're giving yourself time to release your muscular and nervous systems as well as your mind and emotions. Since you're fully supported, your body is inclined to let go, which is restorative and freeing, and your body will remember this sensation when you get up and resume your activities.

Exercises Part 2

There are certain phrases you hear over and over in actor training, and "Be in your body" is a common one. It sounds good, but *how* does one allow that to happen? The following exercises give you practical ways to interpret this instruction.

LET GO OF YOUR BODY

- Stand at your full height, with your feet slightly apart and your arms hanging by your sides.
- Think through your Alexander directions.
- Scan your body for tension. Make note of where you sense any.
- Ask the tension to release.
- Allow your breath to flow easily in and out.

GET OUT OF YOUR HEAD

- Sit in a relatively straight-backed chair, with your back against the back of the chair, your feet on the floor, and your hands in your lap. Allow yourself to sit at your full height.
- Think through your Alexander directions.
- Let your breath flow easily.
- Imagine your head full of air.

- Let yourself rock back and forth on your hip joints.
- Move in a circle from your hip joints. Reverse direction. Move in a figure eight.
- If you catch yourself overthinking, come back to your flow and imagine your head full of air.
- Come to stillness. Remember the mental-physical freedom you found.

BE CENTERED

- Stand at your full height, with your feet slightly apart and your arms hanging by your sides.
- Be aware of the amount of space between the top of your head and your feet.
- Have the intention of lengthening and widening.
- Be aware of the room around you and yourself in it.
- Allow your body, breath, and self to be in tune with what is happening in the room.
- Experiment with taking this sense of yourself into everyday movements: stand and sit, bend, pick things up off the floor, open the door to the room. You don't have to be still to be centered.

GET ENERGIZED

- Stand at your full height, with your feet slightly apart and your arms hanging by your sides. The exercise is best done if you're in an empty or nearly empty room.
- Scan yourself for tension.
- Think through your Alexander directions.
- Let there be a flow of breath, freedom, and energy. Imagine it moving through your body.

- Let that energy take you into walking a few steps forward, then back. Repeat a few times.
- Take this into bigger movements. Jump up and down in place. Run or skip around the room. Swing your arms in large sweeping movement, all with ease and flow.

FIND YOUR CONFIDENCE

- Stand at your full height, with your feet wide apart and your arms hanging by your sides.
- Think through your Alexander directions.
- Exhale as you spread your arms out to each side. Repeat twice.
- Exhale as you come up onto your toes and reach your arms up to the ceiling, leaving your shoulders down. Repeat twice.
- Come back to center and sense yourself open, ready to give and receive.

Primary Exercise

PRESENCE

- Stand outside a room.
- Think through your Alexander directions. Let your breath flow.
- Enter the room. See the whole room.
- Be aware of your inner self as well as your environment.
- Walk around the perimeter of the room, aware of all the space around you.
- Walk into the center of the room.
- Allow yourself to be at your full height and width.
- Stretch your arms out to the sides.
- Walk in a large circle, being aware of the whole room as well as the front, back, and sides of your body.

- As you walk in the circle, sigh three times.
- Let the whole room fill with your awareness.
- Leave the room.
- Reenter the room, retaining the sense of openness you found.
- Walk to the center of the room. Allow yourself be expanded and present.

Presence is one of the things acting teachers talk about a lot. But when you are just beginning to study, the concept can seem elusive. You may be able to recognize it in others, but how do you find it within yourself? Some people might say it's a kind of confidence, but how does one find that without forcing it and coming off as cocky? Presence can encompass many emotional states. It can be striking and almost intimidating, or it can be a quiet, contained thing. This exercise gives you a pragmatic way to balance your focus and attention between your inner self and the outer world. It's taking what's inside you and allowing or inviting those watching to enter your imaginative world. Essentially, presence comes from your being fully present. When you bring that into an audition room or onto a stage, the audience will sit up and take notice.

2 BREATHING

This day I breathèd first ...
SHAKESPEARE, *JULIUS CAESAR*, ACT 5, SCENE 3

Why do we even have to discuss breathing? Don't we all breathe? You breathe when you exercise, sit at the computer, sleep, and generally go about your day. Isn't thinking about breathing a waste of time? The short answer is no. There is no more important topic for the actor than breath.

Don't forget that F. M. Alexander's primary problem was breathing. When he was acting, he tightened his neck, shoulder, and back muscles, which restricted his breathing. His neck tension indirectly caused hoarseness and sometimes even made him lose his voice, a very big challenge for any actor.

Holding your breath and making it shallow can cause all kinds of issues, including:

- a tight throat,
- a tense tongue,
- a restricted jaw,
- an immobile rib cage, and
- a stiff abdomen, which can affect the diaphragm.

All these issues can cause significant problems with speaking, singing, and general communication. Breathing shallowly might manifest itself as a sore throat or a scratchy sound in your voice, or some of your words might get swallowed and go unheard. On the other hand, if you let go and release your breathing, it can help with all these problems. But how do you work on your breath effectively on a daily basis?

There are two main points to remember:

1 *Don't hold your breath.*

2 *Don't let your breath be shallow.*

This may seem obvious. In fact you may have had an acting, singing, or movement teacher tell you not to hold your breath. But even when it's brought to your attention, it can keep happening. Breathing shallowly is less obvious. People can squeeze in a breath in a covert kind of way; they don't even know they're doing it. So you may not be aware that your vocal problems originate with the way you breathe.

To most effectively work with breathing, we have to work with freeing the physical body, because the body is the instrument that creates the breath. Where to begin? Awareness.

Breath Awareness

If you remember only two things about the Alexander Technique, I suggest that they be the following:

1 The Alexander process is one of awareness, inhibition, and direction.

2 Once you think through the Alexander process, you focus on releasing the breath.

You can build these moments of *breath awareness* (see pages 37–38) into your daily routine, at first perhaps five times a day—twice in the morning, once in the afternoon, and twice in the evening. Breath awareness is a positive habit that can support you in your effort to maintain good overall health over the course of your entire life.

Another good place to begin is to have a general sense of how the anatomy of breathing works. I recommend you go online to my colleague Jessica Wolf's website, JessicaWolfArtOfBreathing.com. Go to the "rib animation film" page. You'll see a preview of a fascinating simulation of breathing that Jessica developed with an animator. (A full video of the simulation is available for purchase on Amazon.) First you'll see the skeletal system—the spine, shoulder girdle, rib cage, and pelvis—from the front, back, and sides, which gives you a sense of the way three-dimensional breathing occurs naturally. Then you'll see the movements of the lungs and other organs as they get into the act. The overwhelming effect is to remind you that *breathing is movement.*

YOU ARE YOUR OWN INSTRUMENT

You are your own instrument is a phrase that actors hear often in their training. But what does it mean, exactly? If you are a classical pianist, obviously you are deeply connected to the piano. Having maximum freedom in the breath will help the pianist connect to the piano in an even deeper way and will affect their playing and sound. But there is still a physical separation between the artist and the instrument.

Actors, singers, and dancers are not separate from their instruments: they *are* their instruments. You "play" yourself. Having maximum freedom in your breathing is even more vital for you than it is for instrumentalists. If you have a cold, for example, your instrument has a cold. If you grip your body with tension, your instrument is changed—in fact it's an entirely different shape. Remaining open in your breath flow will help you "tune" your instrument to its optimum level.

Breathing Is Functioning

The **diaphragm** is the primary muscle of breathing. It descends and ascends in as you inhale and exhale. The **intercostal muscles**, located between your ribs, are the secondary muscles of breathing. The ribs gently move out and in as you inhale and exhale. Releasing your rib cage area and midriff—not to mention your whole body—will facilitate a coordinated and efficient way of breathing.

Breathing is also called **respiration**. At its simplest level, it is the process of moving air into and out of the lungs—bringing oxygen into the body and expelling carbon dioxide. The body repeats cycles of inhalation and exhalation, though it may be more useful to think of this as a continuous circle that is never broken. In everyday life this process is controlled automatically by a number of systems in your body. But for the actor, there are many reasons why it's useful to make this unconscious process conscious when it is useful to you.

An obvious example would be if you are acting in a large theater with no microphone or amplification. Especially if there are "dead spots" in the theater—locations where sound gets swallowed up—breathing is even more important. In the past, actors were often instructed to "project" their voices, a potentially unhelpful suggestion because it often leads to pushing and forcing. But using your awareness of the space and your intention, it will be possible for you to fill the space with sound, not through pressure or shouting but through coordination and balance.

Much more than just volume, your breathing also gently powers your articulation, your sense of pitch, your laughter, crying, yawning, and coughing. Most important, it is directly connected to your creative impulses. It's true that there are great actors who breathe somewhat shallowly and still perform well. But for the majority of performers, this is not the case. With the breath restricted, it's harder to connect to your inner life: it is literally harder to feel. So one of the easiest ways to deepen and enrich your acting is to breathe freely, allowing you to easily access your mental and emotional life.

RUNNING OUT OF AIR

Sometimes when people practice their breathing exercises, they feel like they're "running out of air" or they "don't have enough breath." This can also happen when practicing speech and singing. But of course it is rarely literally true that a person runs out of air.

What you're probably feeling instead is physical tension. The body is well calibrated and sophisticated. It automatically will have a sense of how much air you need for each phrase. So don't worry: if you feel short of breath, this often means there is tightness in the diaphragm and/or the rib cage, not that you're going to suffocate. Also, tensing the jaw, tongue, and neck can get in the way of free airflow.

It's common to compress the chest down as air is being expelled during exhalation. Remember to lengthen and widen as you breathe out. This expands the "container" that is your self and helps balance and coordinate your breath. Try placing a hand on your upper chest as you exhale to remind yourself to stay elongated as you breathe. If you feel short of air, cue yourself with the words "release and let go."

Letting Go and Allowing for Flow

So often we unconsciously hold ourselves still, whether standing, walking, bending, or sitting. This inefficient bracing of the body stops or reduces the movement of the rib cage and can restrict the motion of the diaphragm. When you work on freeing up your breathing, I suggest you *don't think about what to do but rather what to undo.*

From childhood, we are often taught that if there is a problem, you have to fix it and, preferably, fix it now. But when you're addressing problems with the body and breathing, it's often better to take an indirect approach. Why? *Because it's human nature to attempt to fix tension with more tension.* For example, when some people catch themselves holding their breath, they start **overbreathing**—forcing air in and out. This will cause tightness of the neck, throat, shoulders, and rib cage, which will in turn restrict the sound of the voice in speaking and singing.

By contrast, using the Alexander concept of inhibition—pausing before the inefficient habit has a chance to take hold—will pave the way for an organic, healthy flow of breath. It's like clearing out a room that has too much stuff in it. Or, to use an unpoetic analogy, it's like unclogging a pipe so water can move through. You don't want to have any obstruction in the way. When you eradicate tension, breathing can flow naturally. Freeing your breath will help you release your body, and releasing your body will help you release your breath. It, too, is a circle.

Why Is Process Important?

The concept of immediate results is pervasive. Many people insist that if you have a clear idea of what you want, if you want it badly enough, and if you work hard enough, you'll get it. But pushing for results in acting causes tension, forcing, and rigidity. On the other hand, paying attention to the step-by-step process involved in achieving your goal will help you get the result you want.

For example, if you're in a scene with a partner, and you're only thinking about yourself and delivering your lines the way you practiced them at home, chances are you won't be "in the moment." You won't be listening to your scene partner effectively, and you may not leave yourself open to spontaneous creative impulses. Alexander called this **end-gaining**—the habit of going after results without paying attention to the process. Using the Alexander Technique to be in touch with your body, your breathing, and your creative impulses will help you in the vital task of being process oriented.

INSIDE OUT VERSUS OUTSIDE IN

Some theater practitioners use the phrases **acting from the inside out** and **acting from the outside in**, though these terms are less common than they were in the past. They refer to two great Western European theater traditions. One is the classical tradition of first addressing a character's outer form, a practice that dates back centuries. This can include deciding what a character looks like, what they wear, what their movement is like, what dialect they speak, and, in certain forms of classical theater, what "type" they may represent. From these externals one can begin to form the internal character.

Another tradition is embodied in the American interpretation of the teachings of Konstantin Stanislavsky (1863–1938)—what used to be called the Method, or **Method acting**. This often refers to the work of Lee Strasberg as well as that of Stella Adler, Uta Hagen, Bobby Lewis, Michael Chekhov, Sanford Meisner, and other prominent acting teachers of the mid- and late twentieth century. In this tradition, the first focus is a character's inner life, or the "truth of the character." Adherents believe that the externals of a character will reveal themselves once the internal life is explored.

Both traditions are to be respected, and practices from both traditions can be useful. But in truth there has always been some overlap between the two. Stella Adler, for example, understood the importance of voice, speech, and honoring the styles of various playwrights. Stanislavsky, too, wrote insightfully about movement, costume, makeup, voice, and speech. Many contemporary actors work from both ends of the spectrum, "outside" and "inside" simultaneously.

For many actors, the demarcation between the two traditions may not be useful. How you breathe and speak is part of who a character is. What a character wears affects how they feel and move. Conversely, a character's inner motives will affect their outward behavior. For me, the inner and the outer are all part of an organic whole and can't be separated. *Characters—and real people—are their bodies, breath, voices, movement, emotions, thoughts, and motivations.* It is a **gestalt**, a word the online *Cambridge Dictionary* defines as "something such as a structure or experience that, when considered as a whole, has qualities that are more than the total of all its parts." Acting theories and exercises—including those in this book— are meant not as ends in themselves but as tools to help actors do their best work.

Intention Affects Your Breath

It's not clear who first said, "Breath is life." This is both literal and metaphorical. We have so many moments when breath is vital to our experience: the moment of birth, the moment we fall in love (when your breath is "taken away"), and special acting moments when everything seems in sync and you can almost feel the audience breathing as one. Your breath responds in various ways to various situations, so its capacity, length, and depth are always changing. In an ideal world, when something happens, we respond first with our breath and then with our whole being.

But sometimes a problem creeps in, and *tension gets in the way.* Tension is often linked with anxiety. There are many theories about nervousness and anxiety and their relationship to performing. It's true that there will probably always be some degree of nerves mixed with excitement when performing. That's fine, and as it should be. But what if your nerves grip your body and your breath and you freeze? What if you find yourself inhibited and not able to perform at your best?

In this situation, it helps to understand why breath is so important in life and in acting:

- Your body responds to your thoughts.
- Your body responds to your emotions.
- Your breath responds to your thoughts.
- Your breath responds to your emotions.
- *If you have a simple, clear intention, you can influence mind, body, and breath.*

THE FIGHT-OR-FLIGHT RESPONSE

The **fight-or-flight response**, also called the **startle response**, is a reaction to a perceived threat. You sense danger, and you tense up. Sometimes you freeze; sometimes you become physically agitated. Several systems in the body respond in a strong way. Some experts say this response evolved thousands of years ago in order to protect humans in the wild. If a person was in a physically dangerous situation, the surge in hormones enabled them to run away or fight.

The trouble is, this doesn't help us in modern-day stressful situations—e.g., when you're running late, caught in traffic, dealing with challenging people, or learning a role on short notice. Your heart pounds, you sweat, your muscles tense, and your breathing becomes shallow and quick. Learning to free your breathing can help in these challenging situations more effectively than the panic that the fight-or-flight response brings. The most important step is to *realize* that you're going into fight-or-flight mode. With practice you'll remember to release the body and release the breath so you can gradually bring yourself out of this state.

So when your nerves get in the way, practice allowing your breath to flow. As you practice, you will learn how intention can affect all your activities.

The *power of habit* in breathing can't be overestimated. A major part of the Alexander process is recognizing the stubbornness of habit.

A component of that is understanding that many unconstructive habits are unconscious, or *below the level of awareness*. Bringing your physical, kinetic, and respiratory habits into your conscious awareness is enlightening. It's not possible to change what you don't know you're doing.

When I was a drama student, my neck was very tight and displaced forward—it wasn't in line with the rest of my body. My shoulders were tight and raised, my arms were squeezed into my torso, and my lower back was markedly arched forward. All these habits affected my breathing adversely. My squeezed neck and shoulders restricted the amount of air I could take in easily, and my tight lower back and rib cage meant that it was difficult for my breath to drop down freely, all the way through my lungs. This meant that my breath was caught in the upper part of my lungs and rib cage. It made my voice slightly breathy and even influenced the pitch, pushing it up slightly.

The Alexander Technique taught me how to loosen the muscles of my neck, which helped them naturally elongate and come in line with the rest of my spine. This improved my head–neck relationship, helping my head balance "forward and up" on top of my spine instead of compressing "back and down." The technique also helped me integrate what was happening in my lower back with the rest of my torso and helped me loosen the intercostal muscles between my ribs. This meant that it became easier for my diaphragm to ascend and descend, and it was easier for my ribs to move in and out. As breathing became significantly easier for me, this changed my voice. It allowed me to find my authentic sound, which was a little deeper, less breathy, and fuller and steadier.

Each of our breath patterns is individual: each of our voices is uniquely our own. That's part of what makes us distinctive as actors. *Changing your unconstructive breathing habits will help you become more yourself.* Whether you are doing an intimate scene in front of a camera or performing on a large outdoor stage in front of hundreds of people, the Alexander Technique can help you find *flow and freedom*.

Everything starts with awareness: giving your attention to the process. The Alexander directions are process instructions to help you make sure you don't leap to the result. Repeating this process just as a dancer repeats *pliés* at the barre will help make the Alexander process organic for you. It will become part of who you are as a person and as an artist.

Let's get to work—in an easy way.

JOURNAL

Keep *a breath journal* for one week. Make a note of whatever stands out to you about your breathing. Write a few words three or four times a day.

1   What do you notice about your breathing in the morning, afternoon, and evening? Is there a difference depending on the time of day?

2   How does your breathing alter with the activity you are doing? Does it seem shallow, deep, or somewhere in between?

3   What happens to your breathing right before you speak?

4   Note if and when you hold your breath throughout the day.

5   When you anticipate a challenging situation, what happens to your breathing?

6   List breath goals for yourself over the course of the next few months.

Exercises

FREEING THE THROAT PART 1

- Stand or sit comfortably.
- Think through your Alexander directions. Allow yourself to be at your full height.
- Let your neck be free three-dimensionally, in the front, back, and sides.
- Allow the inside of your mouth and throat to be easy.
- Yawn as naturally as possible. Allow the mouth and throat to be easy as you do.
- Repeat three more times.

This is a quick and effective remedy for anyone who suffers from performance anxiety (stage fright). A series of yawns tends to soothe the fight-or-flight response; indeed, dogs and cats yawn to calm themselves when they are anxious. In addition, yawning will indirectly help release your jaw and tongue, thus freeing your speech and singing.

FREEING THE THROAT PART 2

- Sit or stand comfortably.
- Think through your Alexander directions. Allow yourself to be at your full height.
- Leave your hands easy as you place them on the front and back of your neck.
- Think of your neck muscles releasing, or melting. Allow your head to be balanced at the top of your spine.
- Remember where the top of your spine is—in between your ears, at the top of your nose.
- Leaving your neck long, look down toward the floor. This will release the back of your neck.
- Slowly return to center.
- Remember the top of the spine as you look up toward the ceiling. This will gently stretch the front of the neck.
- Slowly return to center.

This simple exercise helps release your head at the top of your spine. And it reminds you that your head is never fixed or frozen in one rigid position. Ideally, your head is poised at the top of your spine at all times, ready to move in any direction you want it to go.

BREATH AWARENESS

- Pause briefly as you walk down the street, sit in class, or fix yourself breakfast.
- Ask yourself, "What is happening with my breathing?"

- Scan your body for tension. Pay special attention to your head–neck relationship, shoulders, and torso. You may sometimes catch yourself holding or squeezing your breath.
- Remind yourself that you don't want to stay with your old breathing habits.

RELEASING YOUR BREATH

Let yourself be quiet in body and mind in this exercise. It will help you be more aware.

- While you are in a standing or sitting position, or while you are lying on the floor, place your hands at the bottom of your rib cage on each side. Leave your hands relaxed.
- Do you sense any movement in your rib cage?
- Resist the temptation to "breathe deeply."
- Think through your Alexander directions.
- Tell yourself, "Let go of my ribs. Let my breath flow."

If you sense movement in your rib cage, what kind of movement is it? And is it different on one side or the other? You may not feel any movement, or the movement may be subtle or uneven. The body's tendency is to get used to its own habits. So the feedback you get sometimes may be, "Status quo. All is well," even when the rib cage is rigid or tense.

I asked you not to "breathe deeply" because this would probably encourage your ribs into an overly muscular motion. Because you are standing or sitting quietly, you don't need a lot of air. If, for example, you were running, you would need quite a bit of air, but even then you wouldn't want to take in more than is necessary. You always want the breath to be efficient. Forcing in too much air will result in various kinds of physical tension.

Try this exercise every day for a week. It will take just a minute or two. You may be surprised how much it raises your awareness of your breathing patterns. You'll catch yourself holding your breath at various moments and learn how to let it go.

HOW NERVES AFFECT YOUR BREATH

Some people call easy, quiet breathing a "neutral state." I would call it an open, receptive state. As you become more familiar with this state, you may find yourself less nervous when performing. Allow yourself a minute or two a day to explore this way of being.

- Sit in a relatively straight-backed chair, with your back against the back of the chair, your feet on the floor, and your hands in your lap.
- Think about your head–neck relationship.
- Think through your Alexander directions.
- Think of something that makes you nervous.
- Let that thought go. Return to an open, receptive state.
- Note how your breath shifts.

When thinking of something that makes you nervous, you can imagine having to stand up in front of a large group of people to sing with no preparation. Or having an audition in an hour and needing to memorize a long monologue for it. Or you can think of something that actually happened in your life to make you nervous. When you imagine this, your old habits will probably kick in. You may sense a squeezing in your neck, shoulders, or chest. You may feel yourself holding your breath or tightening your belly or lower back. The body has strong habits that can come to feel "normal" even if they are not good for you. If something is habitual, often the signal you get from your body is that "all is well." But simply asking your breath to be easier and more free can make a marked difference.

FINDING YOUR QUIET, OPEN BREATH

- Lie down on the floor, on your back. Make sure you are lying on an exercise mat, rug, or carpet.
- Place a softcover book or two under your head so that it's raised two to three inches off the floor.
- Bend your knees and place your feet on the floor.

- Put your hands on your lower rib cage.
- Think through your Alexander directions.
- Sense what is happening underneath your hands. Let your mind and body be quiet.
- Have the intention to let your breath be "open" without doing anything to make that happen.
- See if you can allow your ribs to move without forcing them to do so.

As you do this exercise, sense what is happening beneath your hands in your body. Note any movement or lack of movement. Note if the two sides of your body feel different. Allow your breath to flow. See if you can allow your mind and body to be easy and quiet without attempting to hold yourself still. Be aware of the movement of your breath as well as the small movements in your rib cage and in your midsection. You don't need to manipulate your breathing to breathe deeply. Allowing yourself to breathe without obstruction is your objective.

LEARNING ABOUT YOUR BREATHING HABITS

- Stand or sit as you do habitually.
- Read out loud from a book or mobile device. Speak as you do in everyday life.
- After reading for a minute or two, notice what you are doing with your body.
- Note what you are doing with your breath.
- Think through your Alexander directions, then read again.
- See if you can leave your neck free and your head–neck relationship undisturbed.

What happens with your head–neck relationship in this exercise? With your shoulders and back? Also note what's happening with your arms and legs. Are you able to sense what's happening with your rib cage and your abdominal area? Is your breath held or shallow as you read aloud? Is your neck tightening? If you're not sure, place your hands lightly on those areas to collect information. Then see if you're able to read without falling into your old habits.

OBSERVING BABIES AND ANIMALS

- Sit quietly near a human baby or domestic animal, preferably when it is asleep.
- Watch what happens in the nostril area.
- Observe the rib cage moving, from the back and sides if possible.
- If appropriate, gently touch the rib cage to feel the motion of the ribs.

Of course this exercise will depend on your access to children under the age of four and/or domestic animals. (If you don't have access, try looking at extreme-close-up videos online.) You and the child or animal will need to be quiet and calm so as not to interrupt the natural "resting state" breathing pattern. If the child or pet is asleep, that's ideal, since that's when the breath is in its most natural state. From the back, you'll be able to see the free movement of the whole rib cage. Place one hand on the child's ribs and one hand on your own. See if the child's flexibility and elasticity can encourage your own.

OBSERVING GREAT ACTORS

- Choose an actor who is a favorite of yours—contemporary or classic.
- Watch film or video footage of the actor.
- Mute the sound so you can concentrate on the actor's breath.
- Watch how the actor's body moves.
- Pay special attention to what is happening around the nostrils, the jaw, the neck, the rib cage, and the midsection.

People watching is a common exercise given to actors. Usually, the assignment involves watching people going about their activities in public, unaware they are being observed. Students gather information about them and take an almost investigative approach. In this context, the primary focus is how an established actor allows the breath in and out, both when listening and when speaking.

In addition, notice how the breath relates to the rest of the actor's physicality. Can you intuit what the actor's breathing patterns are? Can you determine how much has been changed for the playing of this particular character? Keeping the sound muted, take a few minutes to see if you can imitate what the actor does with their breath.

This is a technical exercise as well as a general acting exercise. The breath pattern will help you *feel* something. *The breath is part of the character's truth.* Observing another actor's breath patterns will help you learn about your own.

HISSING

- Sit in a relatively straight-backed chair, with your back against the back of the chair, your feet on the floor, and your hands in your lap.
- Think through your Alexander directions.
- Release yourself up into your full height and width.
- Tune in to your breathing. Note the gentle movement of your rib cage.
- Let out an extended s sound—a hiss.
- Repeat, a little louder.
- Repeat a third time, a little louder still.

The key to this exercise is to remain easily at your full height and let the air out in a focused and gently controlled manner without getting tight. Let your neck remain easy and the base of your tongue and jaw remain free. Also, see that you don't collapse your chest or tighten your lower back as you hiss.

BLOWING OUT AIR

- Stand one foot away from a full-length mirror. Stand at your full height, with your feet slightly apart. If you don't have access to a full-length mirror, use a hand mirror or bathroom mirror.
- Shape your lips as if you are going to say, "Oh."
- Remaining free in your body, blow out a steady column of air and direct it toward the mirror.
- Repeat, standing two feet away from the mirror.
- Repeat, standing six inches away from the mirror.

You may catch yourself resorting to some unconstructive breathing habits in this exercise. See if you can focus on *allowing* your body to open up as you do it rather than shortening your stature or compressing your chest or shoulders. Have a sense of a free face, lips, jaw, tongue, and body as you breathe out. Make sure not to push. Leaving your body elastic and flexible will help your breath flow freely.

HUMMING

- Sit in a relatively straight-backed chair, with your back against the back of the chair and your feet on the floor. Place your hands easily in your lap, palms resting on your thighs.
- Alternatively, lie down on the floor, on your back. Make sure you are lying on an exercise mat, rug, or carpet. Place a softcover book or two under your head so that it's raised two to three inches off the floor. Bend your knees and place your feet on the floor. Place your hands at your sides.
- Think through your Alexander directions.
- While lengthening and widening, be aware of your breath.
- Think of a simple tune, maybe one you know from childhood.
- Leave your body free and open while humming the tune.
- Notice your breath after you finish humming.

Humming seems primal. It's something we do almost from birth—sometimes consciously, sometimes unconsciously. To hum, we must breathe. The length of the phrases we hum will vary. Your body will make subtle shifts naturally to adapt to the different phrases: it will know how much air to take in. Humming isn't intimidating—as performing Shakespeare can be, for example—so you can easily experiment and have fun with it. The more you can feel "at one" with humming, the easier your breath will be. See if you can retain some of the ease of breath flow from humming throughout the day.

Primary Exercise

WHISPERED "AH"

- Stand with your feet slightly apart and your arms hanging by your sides.
- Allow yourself to stand at your full height.
- Think through your Alexander directions.
- Rest the tip of your tongue easily behind your lower teeth.
- Think of having an inner *Mona Lisa* smile—a small rather than broad smile.
- Breathe out on a whispered "ah" vowel.
- Repeat twice more.

Thinking of having a slight smile helps the breath by releasing facial muscles, including those of the lips, tongue, and jaw. Leaving the tip of your tongue behind your lower teeth allows for an easy opening of your jaw when you breathe out. It's sometimes helpful to have an image of your body as an open column as you breathe out, with no obstruction anywhere along the line. Allowing yourself to be long and wide will help facilitate a free flow of air.

3 YOUR VOICE

O, how wonderful is the human voice! It is indeed the organ of the soul!
HENRY WADSWORTH LONGFELLOW, *HYPERION*, 1839

Just mentioning the voice is enough to make some actors (even famous ones) feel uncomfortable. "I hate the sound of my own voice," "I try never to listen to recordings of myself," and "I wish I sounded different" are common performers' laments. At the other end of the spectrum, there may be a few actors who fall into the trap of *overlistening* to themselves in rehearsal and performance. Whatever your habitual ways of thinking about the subject are, voice training is one of the most vital and fundamental elements of an actor's education. It helps you be heard; it helps you be understood—in both literal and metaphorical ways.

In this book we will discuss the ways in which the body and the voice intersect. By this time it may come as no surprise to you that what is happening in your body affects what is happening in your voice: they are intricately interconnected through the conduit of the breath. One of the best ways to find the full potential of your speaking and singing voice is by freeing and opening your body. I often work in tandem with voice teachers. In this chapter I discuss the physical freedom that can help to free the voice.

In the first chapter I asked, "What do you think a good actor's body is?" Now I will ask, "What do you think a good actor's voice is?" Here's my answer to the question:

- A good actor's voice is one the audience understands.

- A good actor's voice is believable and faithful to any character the actor plays.

- A good actor's voice can sustain itself from curtain to curtain eight times a week.

A related question is, "What is the mechanism that helps create a good actor's voice?" The answer may seem obvious: *you speak from your body and your breath.* The freer your body, the freer your breath and voice. The freer your body, the easier it will be for you to be heard and understood and the more authentic the sound of your voice will be.

Physicality and Your Voice

Let's define the term "**authentic voice**." All bodies are structured a little bit differently. The shape of the head—in particular, the cheekbones, jaw, and tongue—will certainly affect the sound of the voice. The size and shape of the rib cage and back will also have much to do with your unique sound. Your overall size, shape, and body type will all influence your sound. And your sound may subtly change as you get older.

While it's certainly possible for you to alter your sound consciously when you want to or need to, it's helpful to be familiar with your own natural voice before you try to change it. I would define your authentic voice as *coming from your open physical instrument, powered by free-flowing breathing.* This will organically create a sound that vibrates healthfully, with natural overtones and undertones. Whether you're speaking or singing, it's a sound that fills the space you are in without undue effort, and it is connected to the reality of the character you are portraying. Such a voice is easy to listen to and easy to understand. The audience feels the truth of the character viscerally.

Another important point: it's not only your physical structure that helps create your sound, it's also how you *use* that structure. There are many ways that people can unconsciously force their voices, especially at the **vocal onset**, the moment you begin to speak. It's very common for people to tense at the moment of creating sound and speech. Some aspects of the tension may be purely physical: tightening the neck, lifting the shoulders, holding the breath, arching the lower back, even tightening the legs. But there may also be psychological habits that have physical and vocal manifestations. Some people are shy about expressing themselves. Others may be concerned about how they sound and how others may perceive them.

Think of vocalizing as similar to playing a chord on the piano. In playing the piano, you place your fingers on the keys, the hammers inside the piano strike strings, vibrations are created, and those vibrations are amplified by the sounding board and the wood casing of the piano. The end result is what the audience hears. What initiates the human voice is not fingers on keys but rather an electrical impulse from the brain that causes breath to move into the body and out again. When the air passes through the vocal folds, it causes the folds to vibrate. But there is also vibration throughout the whole body, as there is on the wooden casing of the piano.

The vibration that happens in your body may become more resonant over time. This is not because you're attempting to be louder or because you push to make the vibration happen. It's because you make room for it through conscious intention.

How you perceive and evaluate sound—in other words, the sounds you think are pleasant and those you think are unpleasant—may affect how your voice functions. The sound of your family's and close friends' voices will also influence you, as will the part of the country you are from. Many factors intersect with your physical instrument to create your unique sound.

Exploring How Physicality Affects the Voice

I like to assign my students an exercise that I call "Sound Container." To begin, purchase a roll of kraft paper, available at many art supply stores, either bricks-and-mortar or online. You'll need a roll that's at least thirty-six inches wide and seven feet long. Roll the paper out on the floor and lie down on it, then ask a friend or classmate to trace the outline of your body on the paper with a crayon or marker. Stand up and look at the shape that is you, then use the crayon or marker to color in the parts of your body that are important in making sound. Draw the vibrations that represent sound in the places where they come out of your body. After you do the exercise, see the appendix on page 147 for ways you can interpret what you did.

It's also useful to observe the people around you and take note of the way they use their voices in speaking, singing, humming, and so forth. This week, spend a few minutes each day listening closely to the people around you—family, friends, classmates, and strangers. What do you hear? Some may remind you of the way you make your own sound, and others may be quite different from your experience. These comparisons could be useful if you happen to play a character whose voice is similar to one you have heard in daily life.

Also note how the people you observe use body language, gestures, and movement in relation to sound. Do they seem to be in sync or out of sync? Does the body seem to be flowing yet the voice seem staccato? Or is it the opposite? The main point is to be *curious and nonjudgmental.*

The online *Collins Dictionary* defines "nonjudgmental" as "avoiding or tending to avoid making value judgments; tolerant, liberal." When you suspend overly harsh judgments about people's voices, bodies, and behavior, you can feel empathy for them. That is a big part of the actor's job. Empathetic actors will be able to fully embody their roles without "commenting" on the characters. Then they can show the characters in all their complexity rather than giving a surface performance.

Sometimes the most challenging person to withhold judgment from is yourself. But as you work with the exercises in this book you'll become able to observe your habits of breathing, speaking, and physicality without giving yourself a hard time. When you are gentle with yourself, you will learn faster and more efficiently.

LEARNING HOW TO USE VERBAL CUES

Verbal cues—another term for the Alexander concept of direction—are self-generated reminders of your thoughts and intentions. In my experience, the mind and body respond best to words and phrases that are simple, clear, and gentle. If you catch yourself slumping or tensing, for example, it's often not effective to pull yourself up into a rigid military posture. It looks "straight," but a few minutes later, people usually slump back down into their habitual patterns. But the Alexander process of (1) becoming aware of your use in the moment, (2) inhibiting unconstructive habits you don't want, and (3) asking yourself to release your neck, let your head go forward and up, and let your torso lengthen and widen will help your body maintain a tension-free state for a longer period of time and with less effort.

> Rather than admonishing yourself when you catch yourself in old patterns, you can gently remind yourself *what you want* in order to improve. Try talking to yourself the way you would speak to a small child or a close friend. Your body will respond positively to these constructive and encouraging verbal cues.

Staying with Yourself

An important part of practicing any exercise in this book is to, ideally, **stay with yourself**, an important term in the Alexander Technique. It means that you will not lose yourself in what you're doing and that it's possible to stay balanced as you engage in an activity. In other words, you do not need to hold your breath, tense your body, or restrict yourself in any way as you focus on doing something. You can be aware of your body, your breathing, and your thoughts as you carry out an activity. This may seem obvious, but actors "lose themselves" all the time. It's easy to get distracted by the many things that happen in classes, rehearsals, and auditions. But you can balance and coordinate your attention between your inner self, the activity you are doing, and the environment. It may sound challenging, but becomes easier with practice.

One way actors lose themselves is by trying too hard. But *trying harder doesn't always mean you are performing better.* Perhaps instead of exhorting yourself to try harder, you might think about:

- clarifying your objectives,
- drawing up an action plan,
- applying yourself to your plan, but without vocal or physical restriction, and
- revising your objectives and plans whenever necessary.

In addition, when you're listening to the voices of the people around you, you don't need to strain to listen. In fact straining may restrict the amount of sound you can hear and take in. Your objective is to *allow* yourself to hear sounds. You're almost like a scientist gathering data.

Constructive Listening and Observing

It's easier to hear others objectively than it is to hear yourself objectively. But by "objectively," I don't mean without warmth or feeling. I'm simply suggesting that you not jump to conclusions or make quick negative assumptions.

As you listen to others, you'll learn more about your own instrument and how to evaluate what you hear. Another way to hone your listening skills is to choose one or two actors you admire and watch them in films or on YouTube. (The advantage of YouTube is that you can watch videos as many times as you like.) Think through your Alexander directions as you watch. Observe what the actor is doing physically and vocally. How is the voice related to the body, movement, and gestures?

MORE ABOUT THE USE OF THE SELF

We know that "the use of the self" means the ways in which you function mentally, physically, and emotionally in daily life. Among other things, it also means the way you sit, stand, and walk.

But this is very different from the concept of "good posture," which implies a rigidly held stance. Moreover, if we expand our understanding of "use" to include all aspects of ourselves, we can see that the term also applies to the way we use ourselves vocally. In truth, it's not possible to completely separate all the parts of ourselves. For the purposes of an exercise, we might choose to focus on one aspect—breath, voice, body, movement, the mind—but in actuality they are all intricately interconnected. Ultimately we're looking to integrate what we learn in individual exercises into an organic whole. An open mind will help to create an open body. An open body will reinforce an open mind. Free-flowing breath will help both the mind and body. And freeing all these components will help promote easeful, efficient movement and functioning. Which is a fancy way of saying, *If you let go, your acting will improve. And if you continue to let go, your acting will continue to improve.* Ideally, an actor works with this principle for their whole career.

Write down some of your impressions in your journal. Would you say the actor has a distinctive voice? What are the qualities you hear in it? Would you say it's expressive? If so, in what way? How does the actor use voice to communicate?

Does the language of the actor's body seem to be in unison with the voice? If you had to guess, would you say their voice on film is close to their everyday voice, or do you think they have highlighted certain aspects of it for the sake of playing a character? As I suggested in the previous chapter, notice how the breathing, voice, and body are working together. How does that affect the actor's performance in the scene? While some people might say these questions are merely technical, I believe they all relate deeply and profoundly to acting.

Vocal Authenticity Influences Acting Authenticity

We often take the voice for granted. We assume that it will always be there for us whenever we need it. But certainly we are all aware of great speakers, singers, and performers whose voices form an integral part of what they do. Their voices draw the audience in. That's why they do everything they can to maintain their voices by staying open and balanced in every part of themselves.

At this point in your development, it's important to discover what is inherently unique about yourself—that is, to find your own original voice, which originates in your open, released body. That, in turn, will affect your acting deeply.

Use the exercises below to help you to move in this direction.

JOURNAL

1   Keep a voice journal for one week. Note how the way
    you use your body affects your voice. What happens to
    your voice if you tighten your neck, hunch your shoulders,
    or slouch over? How does this affect your breathing

and speech? If you are feeling physically balanced and coordinated, what happens to your voice?

2   Does your voice sound different in certain situations, such as when you're under stress? What about when you are talking to certain people as opposed to others?

3   Take note of what happens to your voice after lying in constructive rest (page 22) for fifteen minutes.

Exercises

RELEASING THE LARYNX

- Lie down on the floor, on your back. Make sure you are lying on an exercise mat, rug, or carpet.
- Place a softcover book or two under your head so that it's raised two to three inches off the floor.
- Bend your knees and place your feet on the floor.
- Put your hands on your lower rib cage.
- Think through your Alexander directions.
- Make sure you aren't gritting your teeth.
- Let your breath flow in and out easily.
- Place your hands quite gently on either side of your larynx.
- Lightly massage the muscles on both side of the larynx.
- Think of the front of the neck and all around the larynx as being loose and free.

In speech and singing, the larynx moves slightly as sounds are formed during **phonation**, the process by which the movement of vocal folds and breath create sound. But often the front of the neck becomes very stiff, and this restricts the subtle movements the larynx needs to make. By freeing up the front of the neck and the area around the larynx, it opens up many possibilities for your voice. You might be surprised by some of the sounds you can make easily when your neck is free.

FREEING THE BASE OF THE TONGUE

- Sit or lie down comfortably.
- Think through your Alexander directions.
- Let your breathing be easy and slow.
- Place two of your fingers, or your thumbs, at the very base of your tongue, just above your larynx.
- Gently massage the base of your tongue, without disturbing the larynx, for one to two minutes.
- Continue to let your body and breath be flexible as you work on the tongue root.

The root of the tongue can be one of the tightest places in the body for many people. This affects voice, speech, and singing. If the base of the tongue is stiff, it presses down on the larynx, which restricts its movement. It can also restrict the sound of the voice. Releasing the tongue can be one of the best ways to help your voice be its freest. If you practice this exercise twice a day for a week, you will sense a real difference in how the tongue functions.

LETTING GO OF THE JAW PART 1

- Sit comfortably.
- Think through your Alexander directions. Allow yourself to lengthen and widen.
- Allow your breath to flow easily in and out.
- Place your fingers on the muscles of the jaw, slightly below the cheekbones, on the sides of your face.
- Gently pulse the muscles to get a sense of how loose or free the muscles might be.
- Massage the jaw muscles in a circular motion.
- Reverse the direction of the circles.

Tension in the jaw can be a pervasive issue for many actors. A tense jaw can affect speech and singing and can even contribute to other problems such as **TMJ** (temporomandibular joint pain). TMJ can result in lockjaw, toothache, and trouble chewing, among other disorders. By contrast, releasing the jaw can have many benefits, including easier breathing. After thinking through your Alexander directions, ask yourself to release your tongue, jaw, and base of the skull to help bring about change in those areas. The more you practice, the more your body will respond.

LETTING GO OF THE JAW PART 2

- Sit or stand comfortably.
- Look in a mirror at your jaw.
- Observe how your jaw opens and closes.
- Place your hand easily on your jaw.
- Use your hand to gently guide your jaw open and closed.
- Use your hand to guide your jaw slowly and easily from side to side.
- Let your hand lead your jaw in a few small circles. Reverse the direction of the circles.

Try to observe the movement of your jaw objectively, almost as though you're looking at someone else. That way it's easier to spot some of your own habits. You may notice that your mouth opens slightly unevenly: it may pull more to one side than the other. Or you might notice that your upper lip stiffens or that your jaw seems somewhat reluctant to open. It's useful to gather this information so you can catch yourself in the act. The freeing of the jaw muscles will help reduce these habits and gradually change them over time.

SOFTENING THE MUSCLES AT THE BASE OF THE SKULL

- Sit in a relatively straight-backed chair, with your back against the back of the chair, your feet on the floor, and your hands in your lap.

- Think through your Alexander directions.
- Place your fingers at the base of your skull.
- Gently explore with your fingers to get a sense of what is happening with those muscles.
- Gently massage the muscles at the base of your skull.
- Easily turn your head from side to side, then up and down.

The muscles at the base of your skull are called the **suboccipital muscles**, which are postural muscles and aid in the movement of the head. It's common for people to be tense here. If you're tight here, it will tense the jaw and tongue.

EASING THE UPPER FACE AND HEAD

- Lie down or sit comfortably.
- Think through your Alexander directions.
- Allow your breath to flow in and out—low and slow.
- Place your palms over your forehead to encourage it to let go.
- Place your palms on your temples, next to your eyes.
- Place your palms over your eyes.
- Put your hands on top of your head, then on the back of your head, to remind those areas to soften.

Releasing the muscles of your face and head—the forehead, the temples, the cheekbones, and the sinus cavities—will help you increase your vocal variety. In this way, there is more richness and nuance in your voice as you speak or sing. More freedom = more overtones = more resonance.

OPENING THROUGH YOUR CHEST

- Lie down on the floor, on your back. Make sure you are lying on an exercise mat, rug, or carpet.
- Place a softcover book or two under your head so that it's raised two to three inches off the floor.
- Bend your knees and place your feet on the floor.

- Spread your arms out wide on either side.
- Let yourself be long and wide. Think about being wide and open through your chest and upper back.
- After a few minutes, if it's comfortable, move your arms above your head, along the floor.
- Place your hands on your upper chest.
- Think about your upper chest softening and opening.
- Allow your breath to flow in and out.

It's not unusual for people to brace themselves and/or collapse through the chest. If the chest is not expanded to its fullest natural dimensions, the breath—and thus the voice—can become blocked or shallow. Rather than pushing your shoulders back or puffing up your chest, it's more effective to allow your upper torso to expand organically, which expands the container through which the breath and energy—and, once again, the voice—of your character can move.

RELEASING THROUGH YOUR RIB CAGE

- Lie down on the floor, on your back. Make sure you are lying on an exercise mat, rug, or carpet.
- Place a softcover book or two under your head so that it's raised two to three inches off the floor.
- Bend your knees and place your feet on the floor.
- Place your hands on your lower rib cage. This will help you remain open through your shoulders and chest.
- Think through your Alexander directions.
- Feel the gentle expansion and contraction of the rib cage as you breathe.
- Silently say the beginning of the alphabet: *a, b, c, d, e, f, g.*
- See if you can leave your whole body free, including your rib cage.
- Say the letters out loud, leaving yourself open as you do so.

When we go from **tidal breathing**—breathing quietly when we're not engaged in vigorous activity—to speaking, often the body feels it needs to do "something extra." Unfortunately, this often means stiffening and tightening. The point of this exercise is to raise your awareness about unconstructive physical habits you may not know you have. It also gives you the opportunity to inhibit those habits. Rather than "doing something" to speak "correctly," you're getting out of your own way, allowing your natural voice to flow out.

PHYSICAL AND VOCAL VIBRATION

- Lie down on the floor, on your back. Make sure you are lying on an exercise mat, rug, or carpet.
- Place a softcover book or two under your head so that it's raised two to three inches off the floor.
- Bend your knees and place your feet on the floor.
- Put your hands on your lower rib cage.
- Think through your Alexander directions.
- Think of your body as an open hollow tube.
- Allow the breath to flow in and out of this tube.
- Hum, initially on one pitch. Then hum on various pitches. Eventually hum a tune, if you wish.
- Allow your body to continue to lengthen and widen.
- Use your hands to feel the vibration throughout your body: face, chest, rib cage, back, and so on.

As you gently place your hands on your face, neck, and chest area, remind yourself that you don't need to force the vibration but rather make room for it to happen. It's a natural occurrence when you don't get in the way with tension, tightening, and forcing. You may be tightening if some areas of yourself are rigid and there is no vibration. But if you do this exercise once in the morning and once in the evening for a week, you'll pick up information about where you may be holding tension, and you'll become more adept at allowing sound to vibrate through your whole body.

BODY INTO SOUND

- Sit in a relatively straight-backed chair, with your back against the back of the chair, your feet on the floor, and your hands in your lap. Allow yourself to sit at your full height.
- Think through your Alexander directions. Allow yourself to release throughout your body 360 degrees.
- Be aware of your breath flowing in and out.
- Blow out through your lips a few times.
- Blow out and let that transition into a hum.
- Blow out again, transition into a hum, then transition into a sustained voiced "ah."
- Repeat twice more.

This simple exercise helps you feel how a released body allows for a released breath. The key is physical freedom. You don't need to do "something extra" when you blow out, hum, or voice an "ah." You want your neck to remain easy, your head to remain balanced and poised at the top of your spine, and your whole body to lengthen and widen. This is the foundation of a healthy and sustainable sound. The quality of the sound is secondary. You might be surprised by what a relief it is not to have to think, "How do I sound?"

TELLING A STORY

- Find a partner or use your phone to record yourself.
- Sit comfortably.
- Think through your Alexander directions.
- Tell a story about yourself—an embarrassing moment, a triumph, or something funny that happened to you.
- After you tell the story, check in with yourself. What happened with your breathing and voice as you spoke?
- If you tightened up, rethink your Alexander directions.

If you really focus on telling the story, you'll most likely be unselfconscious. Depending on the circumstances, you might slip into old vocal habits, or you might be comfortable and easy in your voice. Take note of which it is. If you're not sure, ask your partner to tell you what they heard in a nonjudgmental manner. The objective is to increase your awareness about what you do when you're speaking.

USING YOUR VOICE WITH AN OPEN BODY

In addition to standing on their own, the exercises in this chapter and in Chapter 2 can be used as "after-exercises" in conjunction with the exercises in Chapters 4 through 8. For example, after doing an exercise that addresses movement, resistance, or the mind–body connection, try doing an exercise involving the voice or breathing, such as:

- blowing out air (page 43),
- hissing (page 42),
- the whispered "ah" (page 44),
- humming (page 43),
- releasing through your rib cage (page 56).

Notice what happens to yourself physically as you make sound. What sensations do you feel when you create sound without tension? What happens if you stop worrying about what you sound like?

Primary Exercise

VIBRATION THROUGHOUT YOUR WHOLE BODY

- Find a partner to work with.
- Lie down on the floor, on your back, with your hands at your sides. Make sure you are lying on an exercise mat, rug, or carpet.

- Place a softcover book or two under your head so that it's raised two to three inches off the floor.
- Think through your Alexander directions.
- Hum a series of pitches or a simple song.
- Ask your partner to gently put their hands on various parts of your body to check for vibration. Start at the head, then gently work down to the feet.
- Take note of where there is vibration.
- If there are places where there is no vibration, ask your partner to gently tap on that spot. Notice whether this allows you to release tension there.
- Reverse roles and repeat the exercise.

It's helpful for your partner to gently point out where you have no vibration because it's sometimes easier to feel vibration on someone else than it is on yourself. A gentle touch will help you focus on specific areas. Sensing vibration in your own body will help you become more aware of your use of yourself as a whole. Working on your voice and body are not ends in themselves but important ways you can help develop your artistry and expression.

4 YOUR MOVEMENT

Walk through the gloomy ways of doubt
With the torch of vision in your hand.
ALDOUS HUXLEY, "VISION," FROM *THE BURNING WHEEL*, 1916

Movement is something we often take for granted. Unless you have a disability, physical activities such as walking, sitting, standing, bending, and running are probably relatively easy for you. So why would I devote a chapter to movement? The quick answer is: it will help improve your acting. Consider these scenarios:

- You're standing alone in a very large theater on a steeply raked stage. The only other person on stage with you is the actor playing Titania, who stands on a ladder, which represents a tree. The rest of the stage is empty. You're playing the character of Bottom, who has been turned into a donkey without his knowing it. And you have a scene with Titania in which you have to display the characteristics of a donkey in your body and your voice.

- You're in a film. You stand by the window. The camera frames you in a long tracking shot, which moves in until it becomes a close-up on you. The director has asked you to remain completely motionless. You've been instructed to show the deep pain of losing the person you love, but only with your eyes.

- You're in a play in a tiny black box theater with only forty seats. The play is a comedy, and you've been directed to run and leap around the stage, then suddenly stop, turn, and talk directly to various audience members in an improvisation. Then you have to return to running around the stage, shouting and jumping, then stop to talk to the audience again. And you have to do this several times over.

What you're doing with your body in all these scenarios will make a huge difference in your performance. Ideally, no matter how technically difficult a movement is, you won't want the audience to be aware of the difficulty. Most of the time you want your character's movement to look effortless. Even if you are playing a character who is obviously being physically pushed to the limit—a soldier executing a long series of drills, let's say—it should look like the *character* is being pushed to the limit, not *you*, the actor.

Body Communication

So much communication in life—and in theater and film—is nonverbal. Body language, physical behavior, facial expressions, posture, gestures, eye movements, and the way you occupy space express so much. In plays, TV, and film, actors must convey their objectives through these means, which is why the study of movement in various forms is one of the basic aspects of actor training. And integrating movement with other aspects of the actor's craft is vital—not as an end in itself but rather in service of the character you're playing.

How to ensure that your movement enhances rather than obstructs your performance? Through *coordination, flexibility, strength, and psychophysical intelligence*. Let me define these terms as I use them.

- **Coordination**: Managing the various parts of your body in a smooth and efficient manner so they work as a harmonious whole.

- **Flexibility:** Using your body in a pliable and elastic way to allow for the freest possible range of movement, maximum lengthening, and healthful muscle tone.

- **Strength:** Finding power and potency, vigor and vitality, in your self while maintaining these states over a period of time.

- **Psychophysical intelligence:** Understanding—on an ongoing, developing basis—the ways in which mind and body work in unison to achieve the best possible functioning of the self.

These terms apply to both mental and physical qualities. If you can cultivate them within the full range of your self, you will be in a very good place to do your acting work.

Walking

Most of us don't think about the way we walk, but when I'm coaching someone in a role, one of the first things I ask is, "How do you think your character might walk?" And often the answer is, "I don't know." Then we explore it.

In working with your own movement, the best place to start is by taking stock. Ask yourself what you're doing when you're walking, specifically:

- Which part of your body initiates walking?
- What's happening in your head, neck, and shoulders when you walk?
- What's going on in your lower back when you walk?
- What's happening with your breathing as you walk?
- Are you aware of the movement in all the joints of your legs—hips, knees, ankles, and feet?

Some people initiate walking by pressing the head back and down toward the shoulders. Others pull the neck forward as they begin to walk. Sometimes the shoulders get lifted or rounded forward. The lower back may arch; breathing may get held. Ironically, the joints in the legs may stiffen, which makes walking more difficult.

Thinking the simple idea of lengthening *up* helps coordinate all your body parts. (In fact you can apply this thought to all movements in your daily life: sitting, standing, bending, twisting, lunging, running.) As you lengthen and widen your body, it will lessen tensions such as tightening your shoulders or arching your lower back. And, as I've mentioned, releasing the body always helps to release and open up the breathing.

As you're walking, exercise your **psychophysical intelligence**. Ask yourself what you're doing with your body, your mind, and your breathing. Observe yourself almost as you would a friend—*nonjudgmentally*. Sometimes using a mirror is helpful. As you observe yourself and others, you will hone your observational powers: you'll notice subtle things that make a real difference over time.

Poise and Balance

Two other terms I use when coaching actors in movement are **poise** and **balance**.

- Poise means you're not falling prey to old, unconstructive habits, either mental or physical. It means giving yourself space to inhibit your habitual reactions to stimuli, which gives you time to think through your Alexander directions ("to direct"). It gives you choices in your behavior.

- Balance can be defined as a state in which anything extraneous (e.g., tension) is absent, allowing your natural way of being to emerge. It is a state of efficient equilibrium. It doesn't mean you have to be slow and quiet—sometimes actors need to be loud and quick—but you can do whatever it is you want to do with *an inner steadiness, even in the midst of great activity.*

YOUR BODY WHILE TEXTING

What happens to your body when you text? You've probably seen it in other people: the whole body slumps down to get closer to the device. You yourself may have already heard the suggestion to hold the device higher. But that's not quite enough. If you're still slumped down while holding the device higher, that's not going to help. Use your Alexander directions to help yourself up into your fullest natural height. Then from there, try holding your device higher so your whole body doesn't pull down to it. Try pivoting your head from the top of your spine—up between your ears, behind your nose—allowing your neck to be long as you look down at your device. You don't want to drop your head heavily toward it, putting pressure on your neck and shoulders. See if you can type without tightening your fingers or thumbs. Do one of your breathing exercises from chapter 2, then send a text. Did it make a difference?

Apparent Stillness

Even in the stillness, the movement of your breath continues. In fact, because of this, the very term "stillness" (a state that many acting teachers and directors ask for) may be misleading. It may be more accurate to use the term **apparent stillness**, meaning you *appear to be still to the observing eye* but inside, your breath is moving in and out, your blood is flowing, and you are making infinitesimal movements.

There are many times in a play when it is quite powerful to use apparent stillness—and in film it's necessary and effective much of the time. When you are "still" on film, especially in a close-up, the audience can focus on what the character is thinking and feeling rather than on extraneous movements, no matter how small. Again, stillness does not mean holding your breath and tightening your muscles to lock yourself in place. Rather it's a pause, or a suspension; it's a choice to let go of anything extraneous. So stillness can be a moment in which you let go of anything that isn't necessary. It's an unusual moment, one that is inherently dramatic.

The Startle Response and Neuromuscular Reeducation

For most able-bodied people, sitting and standing are easy—movements they never think about. We all sit and stand dozens of times a day. But what if we do it in a way that is unconstructive or even harmful? It's very common for people to unconsciously have a low-grade fight-or-flight response (also called the **startle response**; see page 34) to these and other everyday movements. It's no wonder: many of us are overscheduled, overstressed, in a hurry, and just plain old creatures of habit. That's enough to set off a startle response.

If you watch people in a public place, you'll see them drop or almost throw themselves into chairs all the time. There's very little control of the movement. When people get up out of their chairs, they're often "hauling themselves up." There is a lot of tension involved with both motions. But it doesn't have to be that way.

WALKING, SITTING, AND STANDING

- Stand across the room from a chair.
- Walk across the room and sit down without thinking about it.

- Stand up in your usual way, then walk back across the room.
- What did you notice? Where did you tense up? Did you hold your breath?
- If you're not sure what you did, repeat this sequence a few times.
- Think through your Alexander directions, then repeat the above series of movements.
- What was the difference?

The online *Cambridge Dictionary* defines "momentum" as "the force that keeps an object moving or keeps an event developing after it has started." In the case of standing up, this may mean that moving a bit faster will help you get up more easily and with a bit less leaning forward, as long as *you keep allowing your head–neck relationship to be balanced. Your head leads, and your body follows.* If you find it challenging in the beginning to get up at a normal pace and not pull your head back and down or arch your lower back, then stand a little bit more slowly when practicing. As you gain experience, you'll be able to use momentum successfully.

As a reminder, the Alexander Technique is not about "having good posture." Rather, it's about *having efficient and graceful movement and balance.* Do your best not to unconsciously tighten up in efforts to "be straighter." When working on your movement habits, it may be inevitable that you overcorrect on the one hand and fall back into your old habits on the other. *This is normal.* But the more you are aware, and the more you focus on the use of your self, the more adept you will become at developing a way of moving that works for you as well as for the characters you're playing.

Being aware of the use of the self as you go about your daily life is what the well-known English novelist Aldous Huxley (*Brave New World*) called "*thinking in activity.*" Another way to characterize the Alexander Technique is as a system of **neuromuscular reeducation**, which is a fancy way of saying that in the Alexander Technique, you use your sensory awareness to work with your muscles and nervous system to improve balance, coordination, and movement.

But this doesn't mean being self-conscious or being "trapped in your head." It means using your brain in daily life and when you're working on your character at home. When it comes to performance, you won't need to think about your physical life so specifically because it's been part of your practice throughout the rehearsal process. *It will organically be there.* You won't need to prove to the director or audience that you've "done your homework."

FOUNTAIN IMAGE

It's sometimes useful to think about *the energy of the body flowing upward*—like water flowing up in a fountain. You've probably seen fountains that gently spray water upward from a spout in a pond or pool. Sometimes the water fans out in all directions. Try thinking about your body that way. Rather than slouching down or holding yourself up, picture yourself as being that small fountain. There is a consistent flow, a movement that is constantly being renewed, and nothing is held. Then think of taking that flowing energy into your everyday activities: walking, running, working out at the gym, sitting at the computer—any of the many activities you take part in during the day.

Overconcentration and Expanded Awareness

F. M. Alexander said, "*The hardest thing to remember is to remember.*" We get so pulled into what we are doing that we forget about ourselves. For example, many of us are taught from a young age to *concentrate*. There are many interpretations of what this could mean. But often it can lead to a kind of **overconcentration**, a kind of hyperfocus on one thing to the exclusion of all else, which sometimes involves holding the breath and tightening the body. This is counterproductive and restrictive to movement, acting, and creativity in general. It is the opposite of a *sense of play*, which is so important in creativity.

I find the concept of **focus** more useful. We can define focus as consciously giving your attention to a task without undue tightness or mental or physical restriction. There is instead an **expanded field of awareness**, which allows you to become aware of stimuli without being overly distracted by them. In the Alexander Technique, as in meditation, if you find your mind wanders too far from what you are doing, you can gently guide it back without straining or forcing.

Throughout this chapter we've considered everyday movements and tasks. These are the building blocks: when you study dance, clown work, masks, commedia, gymnastics, or stage combat, you will have a head start because you've considered and worked with these movement fundamentals.

Movement is a major part of our daily functioning—in a way, it *is* our daily functioning. Allowing it to be a little bit more conscious, a little more mindful, makes all movement easier.

JOURNAL

1   This week, write a list of what you notice about your own movement. Try to be objective, the way you would be about a good friend. Choose various activities from your day and describe your observations about the way you move as you do them.

2   Make a list of actors, well known or otherwise, who move in a way that you admire. What is it about their physicality that you like? Is there anything you can develop in yourself that they have?

3   Bring your journal with you throughout one entire day. Pause in the midst of an activity twice in the morning, twice in the afternoon, and twice in the evening. During the pause, observe your body and physicality. Write down whatever you notice.

Exercises

WALKING

- Stand comfortably.
- Walk across the room as you normally do.
- Pause at the other end of the room. Did you notice anything about your movement?
- Walk across the room again, paying attention to how you move.
- Pause, taking note of whatever stood out to you.
- Think through your Alexander directions.
- Walk across the room again, thinking of an upward direction as you walk.

SITTING

- Stand in front of a chair.
- Sit the way you usually do.
- Then stand the way you habitually do.
- Pause. What happened in your body? What happened in your head–neck relationship? What happened in your shoulders, back, and legs? What happened with your breathing?
- If you're not sure, do it again and take note.
- Now think through your Alexander directions.
- Sit, then stand.
- What was the difference?

SITTING EFFICIENTLY

- Sit in a straight-backed chair, near the front edge. Have your feet flat on the floor, close to the chair.
- Think through your Alexander directions.
- Move forward from your hip joints. Let your head lead and your body follow. Your body stays elongated as you move.

- When your head is over your feet, press your feet down to unfold your legs and come to a standing position.
- Come up into your full height.
- Reverse this to sit down. Lengthen up as you allow yourself to bend at the ankles, knees, and hips. Lengthen yourself into the chair.

The challenge in this exercise is to resist stiffening, or "pulling yourself up," at the beginning. When you come back into the chair, see if you can find a "neutral" place, meaning neither slumping nor rigidly upright. Try folding yourself easily at all the leg joints, as if you were folding a fan. Aim to rest on the sitting bones, or the ischial tuberosity—the base of the pelvis. That helps you remain balanced as you sit. You're looking to be released and lengthened but also energized.

SITTING AT THE COMPUTER

- Sit at your computer, as you would habitually.
- Imagine you are tired and have been sitting for a couple of hours.
- Note what happens in your body: what is the shape of your spine at that moment? What's happening with your head–neck relationship, your shoulders, and your breathing?
- Stand and walk away from the computer.
- Sit again. This time think about lengthening up. Note the ergonomics of your relationship to the keyboard. Lean forward from your hips, if necessary.
- Leave yourself lengthened as you type.

BENDING

- Stand behind a chair with your feet a bit apart.
- Think through your Alexander directions.
- Place your hands at your hip sockets, at the fold where your legs meet your torso.

- Bend your knees forward and lean forward from your hip joints. Rest your hands on the back of the chair.
- Check that you don't pull your head back and down and don't hold your breath.
- Return to standing by straightening your legs. Come all the way up to your full height.

When you are bent forward from the hips, you are in what is called a **position of mechanical advantage**, or the **monkey position**. In leaning forward, aim to neither slouch over from your waist nor to overarch your back. Rather, bend from your hip joints, which helps lengthen your spine and release your breath all the way through your lungs.

Standing in this position with your hands on the back of the chair is a good time to practice the whispered "ah" (page 44). The monkey position is also an ideal way to lean over the bathroom sink when brushing your teeth and to bend down when you want to pick up something heavy. The small joints of the spine are meant primarily for flexibility; the joints of the legs are primarily weight-bearing. Bending from the hip sockets puts most of the work in the leg muscles, where it belongs.

LUNGING

- Bring yourself into a position of mechanical advantage (above) with your hands resting on the back of a chair.
- Let your right leg extend behind you. You are now in a lunge, as you would be in fencing.
- Alternatively, stand a bit away from the chair and step forward with your left foot, so your left knee is bent and your right leg is straight. Your right foot stays completely against the floor.
- Check that you don't pull your head back and down and don't hold your breath.
- Have a sense of how long and wide you are in this physical stance.
- Reverse the position of your legs so your left leg is extended straight behind you and the right knee is bent.
- Notice whether anything feels different once you have switched sides.

There are many instances when bending both knees may not be practical—for example, when vacuuming, pushing something heavy, or bending to reach for something far away. In these instances, lunging can be useful. It is a particularly powerful position of mechanical advantage and one of the positions in which your back will be at its strongest.

HOW TO TEXT

- Stand or sit comfortably.
- Take out your mobile device.
- Don't think through your Alexander directions. Hold your device as you do normally.
- Type a text.
- Pause. Notice what you're doing with your body. What's happening with your head–neck relationship? What's happening in your shoulders, spine, and arms?
- Note where you are holding your device.
- Think through your Alexander directions.
- See what happens if you hold your device higher than you're used to.
- Text again.

USING STAIRS

- Find a flight of stairs.
- Go up and down the stairs in your habitual way.
- Notice your habits: do you slump or lean far over? Do you grip the handrail?
- Go up and down the stairs again, staying with your Alexander directions.
- As you go up the stairs, think of the head leading your spine up.
- As you go down the stairs, think of traveling back and up in space as your knee comes forward.

Thinking back and up when you descend the stairs will prevent a forceful downward pull through your torso. Just because you are going in a downward direction doesn't mean you need to collapse your body. Each downward step can be a reminder to lengthen up. Similarly, going in an upward direction doesn't mean you need to hike yourself up through the neck and shoulders: allow your legs to do the work. Many people mention they feel lighter and easier when they take stairs in this way.

RAISING BOTH ARMS

- Stand comfortably.
- Think through your Alexander directions.
- Slowly raise your arms to the ceiling, imagining that your fingertips are leading the way.
- Your arms are fully stretched up toward the ceiling. Your spine is long. Your shoulders should remain down.
- Continue to think of length and width as you float your arms down.
- Repeat two more times.

Your habit may be to pull your head back when raising your arms. Another thing to watch for is arching through the lower back and/ or pulling your rib cage forward. This may also happen when you use your arms in sports or as you lift weights. Your back will be stronger and more flexible if you leave your upper and lower back integrated, without breaking at the lower back or rib cage.

LOOKING UP AND DOWN

- Stand comfortably.
- Think through your Alexander directions.
- Place your forefingers against each ear.
- Think of an imaginary bar going horizontally through your head at the level of your forefingers.
- Pivot your head to look down. Check that your head doesn't collapse or press onto your neck.

- Return to the central position.
- Look up toward the ceiling. As your head tilts back, imagine it not compressing down onto the imaginary bar.
- Return to the center position.
- Repeat twice more.

We don't want the head to ever be locked in place. Think of it as being easily balanced at the top of your spine: that will help you lengthen through your whole body. There are many times during the day when we need to look up or down, and it's amazing how little we notice about our physical habits as we do so. This exercise will help you increase your awareness and maintain your poise as you do it.

CARRYING BAGS

- Pick up the bag that you carry most often, whether a purse, tote, backpack, messenger bag, dance bag, or gym bag, and put it over your shoulder or onto your back—whichever way you usually walk with it.
- Walk around the room, noticing your physical habits.
- Stand and sit a few times.
- Pick up and put down your bag, taking it on and off your shoulder or back, observing how you manage it.
- Think through your Alexander directions.
- Repeat some of these movements, noticing whether thoughts of lengthening and widening lighten the burden.

Every actor has a bag. Almost every person who lives in a walkable town or city carries a bag. There are pros and cons to various types of bags: one type is not innately better than another. But one of the most important factors to consider is minimalism. Remove everything from your bag that isn't essential, and you'll do your body a favor. Also, carry the smallest bag that is practical. That way you won't stuff it with too many things. If your wear a backpack, avoid the temptation to hunch your body forward as you walk. If you carry a bag on one side, try not to let it pull you down on that side. Switch back and forth between your two hands as you carry the bag.

APPARENT STILLNESS

- Stand or sit comfortably.
- Remind yourself not to lock your joints or stiffen your eyes.
- Let your breath flow in and out easily.
- Think through your Alexander directions.
- Allow yourself to be apparently still for one to two minutes.
- If it helps you, remind yourself of your directions occasionally.

There are many times when a director might ask you to be "still." But don't let this suggestion lead you to *freeze in place*. It's often powerful on film for the actor to "do less." But this doesn't mean going rigid or limp. There is still an *inner aliveness*—you will still have thoughts and feelings and intentions. You have inner action even as you have outer apparent stillness.

THE HUMAN X

- Stand comfortably, feet easily apart, arms at your sides.
- Think through your Alexander directions.
- Spread your feet apart into a wide stance.
- Float your arms up toward the ceiling, into an open V position. Your shoulders stay down. Your body is now like a large X.
- Gently stretch your arms up and out. Tell your whole torso to be long and expanded.
- Float your arms down.
- Repeat the exercise.

This exercise gives you a wonderful stretch through the whole body. You can think of your legs stretching down toward the ground while your arms stretch up toward the ceiling. It's almost as though you are a piece of elastic being gently elongated in two directions. As always when raising your arms, check that you don't arch your lower back or pull your rib cage forward. Remain an integrated, dynamic whole. You can apply these principles to all kinds of active movements in sports and at the gym.

RUNNING

- First observe the way you run habitually, whether outside, in a large rehearsal room, or on a treadmill. What happens with your head–neck relationship, your shoulders, your lower back, and your breathing?
- Speed up, then slow down to determine whether speed affects your habits.
- Pause. Think through your Alexander directions.
- Run again, this time thinking about an upward flow through your torso. Keep your head balanced at the top of your spine. Keep your shoulders easy and open. As your knees come forward, come down evenly on your feet.

When you pause in the midst of an activity to think through your Alexander directions, you are taking a moment to **redirect**—i.e., renew your intentions in a nonjudgmental way. For example, it's tempting to pull your neck and shoulders forward while running. Thinking of releasing in an upward direction will help you counteract that tendency. *The head leads, and the body follows.* The body flows up, and the knees come forward so there is a natural and dynamic two-way stretch. Allowing the breath to flow in and out freely and allowing an easy rotation in the shoulders and hips will help keep running pleasurable and efficient.

Primary Exercise

YOUR CHARACTER'S MOVEMENT

- Choose a character to work on.
- Read the play. Be familiar with the story and the character.
- Stand at your full height, arms easily at your sides.
- Think about the character. Answer these questions:
  - How old is the character?
  - Does the character have the same body type as you do?
  - Is the character's social status different from yours?

- o Does the character move quickly or slowly? Fluidly or sharply? Does the character tread lightly or heavily?
- Keeping the answers in mind, begin to walk.
- Allow the character's age, body type, status, and gait to affect the way you move.
- Take the character's qualities into other movements: standing, sitting, bending, picking things up and putting them down.

It's helpful to work on each of the characteristics mentioned above one at a time. For example, walk back and forth across the room being aware of the character's age. Then add in the body type, walking back and forth a few times; then add the next element, and so on. Spending five minutes or so with this exercise may surprise you with the difference in your own movement. You don't need to "demonstrate" who the character is. *Allow the elements to affect you from the inside.* Who the character is will be reflected in your body and how you use it. That way you won't use clichéd movements: you'll discover unique characteristics that will ring true for the audience.

If your character needs to slouch, rather than slouching down in your habitual way, getting heavy in your body and restricting your voice, allow your body be lengthened into a C curve, thinking through your Alexander directions as you do so. Even though it looks to the audience like you're hunched over, you're not putting unnecessary pressure on your throat, lungs and back. You take the shape of the character without taking on their tension.

5 MENTAL AND PHYSICAL RESISTANCE

High to the blissful wonders of the skies
Elate thy soul, and raise thy wishful eyes.

PHILLIS WHEATLEY, "TO S. M., A YOUNG
AFRICAN PAINTER, ON SEEING HIS WORKS,"
FROM *POEMS ON VARIOUS SUBJECTS,*
***RELIGIOUS AND MORAL*, 1773**

The self-help author Barbara Sher rose to fame in her field with her advice "Do what you love" and "Live the life you love." These exhortations have now been adopted into American culture. But what if you can't seem to do what you love? What if it scares you too much? What if you're a perfectionist, so you never really start because your standards are so high? Or what if you're a person who has no idea where to start?

Barbara won't mind if I share a bit of her personal story. (She's a friend of mine. You can check out her TEDx talk "Isolation Is the Dream Killer," which has more than a million views.) As Barbara often says, if she can go after her dreams, anybody can. At one point she was a divorced single mom with two young boys and no money. She moved to New York City back when it was dirty and dangerous. She did not have a fancy advanced degree; she had no industry contacts, and she wasn't particularly "disciplined." And yet she made a very successful life for herself as a career coach and as the author of a number of bestselling books about creating your own best life. She's especially well known in China, Russia, and Eastern Europe, where these are new ideas.

Start a Creative Support Group

Barbara's main point is that *none of us can do it alone.* This is contrary to the great American myth of "rugged individualism." What we actually need to develop fulfilling lives is to surround ourselves with a group of nonjudgmental, helpful, and positive friends. It's a very simple idea. Other experts have written about certain aspects of her theory, but I've never seen anyone other than Barbara lay it out so simply and comprehensively.

Start thinking about surrounding yourself with a group of people you like and respect and are helpful to you. It's not a one-way street: you'll be helping each other. The size of the group doesn't really matter. Maybe it will be fairly large, or maybe it will comprise just three or four people you can really count on. The main thing is to have their support and to be supportive to them in return.

Perhaps the people in your group will be other actors. Maybe they will be stage managers, designers, playwrights, or theater managers. Maybe they won't be in the performing arts at all. Your group might be multidisciplinary: it might include poets, painters, novelists, or even businesspeople or lawyers who are interested in the arts. The point is that you are all interested in learning and growing, and you're in it together. To paraphrase Barbara, being alone can be a little scary; being in a group that believes in you can make you brave.

Having the support of a group is important, because all of us encounter blocks from time to time. The group will help you when the going gets rough, and it will help when you come up against resistance.

Meeting Resistance

Are any of these resistance scenarios familiar to you?

- You know you should study for a test, but you tell yourself you're just going to scroll on social media for ten minutes. (Which turns into two hours.)

- You want to practice singing each day for half an hour, but you never seem to get to it.

- You have to learn a scene for acting class. You have a week to learn it, but you don't start reading it until the night before, or even right before class. You justify this by telling yourself you're a better actor when you're "spontaneous." (Your teacher may not agree.)

- You delay watching films, seeing plays, and reading books because you're "too busy."

- You'd like to work on the Alexander Technique, but you can't find the time.

If you relate to a few or a lot of these: *don't worry.* These issues are very common. Why? Because **resistance** is a habit ingrained in all of us.

According to the online *Collins Dictionary*, "Resistance to something such as a change or a new idea is a refusal to accept it." Possibly the most important word in that sentence is "refusal." Often our refusal is unconscious. I include myself in this; I've experienced lots of resistance! In fact I have just as much resistance as most people do—possibly more. *But I've learned to work with my resistance, not against it.*

People don't *intend* to resist. For example, there are all kinds of things that are good for us—getting enough sleep, exercising, eating well, and developing good use of the body. We don't say, "Anything that is good for me I'm going to ignore!" And yet we come up with ways to avoid them. What are some of your reasons?

- You think you don't have enough time.

- You mean to do it but keep putting it off.

- You feel scattered and can't focus for any length of time.

- You're involved in so many projects that it's hard to get to anything else.

- You're not sure how to prioritize your "to do" list.

- You have a sense that "I shouldn't have to work for it—it should just come to me."

- You have the philosophy, "If the Universe wants me to have it, it will come."

- Anxiety.

- Fear of failure.

- Fear of success.

- Fear in general.

Fear and Anxiety

Anxiety and fear sound almost melodramatic—could resistance really be related to them? Sometimes it's a very low level of anxiety and fear that contributes to resistance—so low we're not even aware of it. And at other times we do know, very clearly.

There are direct physical ramifications of anxiety and fear. Holding the breath, breathing shallowly, tightening the neck, pulling the head back and down, tensing the shoulders, and squeezing the lower back and legs are all very common. *Our psychology is reflected in our bodies.*

When I was a boy, I loved to swim, and I was good at it. And I did well diving from the low board. But the high board? I'm not afraid of heights, but there was something about climbing the ladder of the high board, standing on the edge, and looking down at the water far below that really frightened me. I knew nothing bad would happen to me when I jumped off the board—I knew the water would buffer me. But I still feared jumping off a board that high.

There are a number of things we encounter each day that can make us anxious or frightened, even if only a little. For example, consider these possible fears:

- Where did I put my keys?
- Did I leave the stove on?
- I hope I'm going to pass that test!
- Does that person really like me?
- Do my teachers like my work?
- Is my acting/writing/directing any good?
- What's going to happen to me when I start auditioning professionally?

Avoiding what scares us keeps our fear level down. But what if you love acting and it scares you on some level? You don't want to avoid acting, but you may postpone learning your lines, procrastinate about planning your course schedule, and avoid certain classes or performance situations because these activities would bring you up against your fear. These actions may be taken unconsciously or partly consciously. But becoming aware of your anxiety and fear, though uncomfortable, is important. It will help you do the things you want to do.

Stress in the Body

Mental and emotional stress get lodged in the body. This is called **somatizing**. Somatizing happens when we do not fully process stress, fear, or anxiety and the body holds on to them physically. By "fully process," I mean work through them mentally and emotionally, deliberately and in detail. As a result, your body attempts to do the processing—a situation that for most of us translates emotional stress into physical tension. To make things more complicated, *we're not always aware when we are stressed.*

Something in our DNA tells us to be safe by avoiding things that are outside our comfort zone. But *performing takes us outside our comfort zone all the time.* So it serves us well to observe and question our own resistance.

In my own case, my past Achilles' heels were my neck, shoulders, and lower back. Paradoxically, my body was attempting to control my stress through tension. I may also have been unconsciously trying to make my body feel more "stable." But my habits only resulted in a much tighter and more restricted body. I repeated this pattern for many years.

Then I learned that *the Alexander Technique is a powerful tool, not just for easeful and efficient movement and functioning but also for the reduction and management of fear and anxiety.*

Fear can be a habit, like anything else. The Alexander Technique teaches us that when you catch yourself in the midst of it, you can become aware of what is happening, decide you want to look at the situation differently, and give yourself verbal cues that will help you discover new behaviors. Over time, with patience and practice, you can find your way out of your fear.

HABIT

A habit is a behavior we repeat often, mostly without thinking. Many habits are beneficial and save us time. For example, you have a certain way of getting dressed and fixing breakfast in the morning. You have a favorite way of getting to school. You developed these habits because they save time and effort—in other words, you don't have to think about any of the many dozens of small movements involved in getting out of bed, getting dressed, eating breakfast, and getting to school. You can do them without thinking.

However, other habits are not necessarily helpful: staying in bed too long, then rushing to get dressed, picking up some poor-quality breakfast food on the way to school, slouching for hours at the computer. Even though you obviously know how to get up out of bed, make toast in the kitchen, and sit at the computer, the *process*, or way you do the activity, could improve. That's where the Alexander Technique comes in. Awareness helps us realize what we're doing, inhibiting helps us stop the bad habit, and directions help us change the habit.

Procrastination

We all procrastinate sometimes—I know I do! There are so many reasons for it: we may think a task is unpleasant; it may not be at the top of our priority list; we may dread it; the task may confuse us and we may not know how to tackle it. And when thinking about something we don't want to do but know we should, we sometimes feel bad about ourselves, which may encourage us to procrastinate even more. Our bodies will be affected by all this.

In fact, your body may sometimes resist your Alexander directions, and *this is normal*. Physical habits, even if they hurt, are on some level comfortable. That is part of what a habit is—it feels normal. But what feels normal may not be good for us and may not even be natural. For example, an easily upright stance is actually normal. You can see infants and very young children in this organically elongated and balanced state all the time. But if slouching and pulling heavily down becomes habitual for you, it can become your "new neutral," which is not really neutral. Sometimes your body may rebel against freeing up, releasing, and sensing a new way of being, a new way of functioning. But I consider this part of the process. *Once your body has experienced physical freedom, it will probably want to return to it as soon as it can.*

For example, everyone knows what it is to slump. You don't have to practice to do it; you can do it immediately. It may feel good for short periods of time because you're so used to it. But if you sit that way for long, you may be begin to feel uncomfortable.

The way I see it, the easiest choice is the most healthful choice: an upward flow of energy through the torso, with your head balanced forward and up on top of your spine and your arms and legs releasing easily away from your torso. If you keep this principle in mind when you feel temporary mental or physical resistance, you'll know that you can always return to the Alexander way of being, which is simply another way of saying the way we are designed to be.

JOURNAL

1   Take five minutes each morning when you get up to write about the resistances you felt the day before or that morning. They can be mental, physical, or emotional. At the end of the week, review your entries and see if you notice any patterns.

2   Write about resistances you sense when engaging in purely physical activities: working out, running, walking, dancing, cycling, and so on. Do you get tight when you resist doing these activities? Do you know why you may resist these activities?

3   Write about any resistance you may have toward the Alexander Technique and its principles. Some people are reluctant to raise their awareness. Others don't like to give themselves verbal cues. What might your resistances be?

Exercises

RESISTING ALEXANDER TECHNIQUE

- Sit or stand comfortably.
- Imagine it's one of those days when you're "just not having it." You don't want to think about your head–neck relationship or the use of yourself.
- Slump down on purpose.

- Make your breath shallow on purpose.
- Pull into yourself. Maybe even feel defensive.
- Ask yourself what this feels like physically.

We all have days that feel a bit overwhelming. Or maybe you feel tired and not quite able to cope in your usual way. You may have many things to do. Any of these situations may lead you to resist thinking about your use of the self. It may be slightly annoying to feel you need to think about it. Perhaps you may even feel a little contrarian about it: "Why do I need to think about this Alexander stuff, anyway?" It's okay. You don't need to force yourself to work on Alexander all the time. But it might be useful to notice what happens to your body when you're in this state.

NAMING IT

- Sit comfortably.
- Remember class or performance situations in which you felt awkward or uncomfortable.
- See if you can put yourself back in that situation.
- Place your hand on your chest.
- Listen to what you're sensing in your body and yourself as a whole.
- Name what you're sensing.
- Breathe out and let the exercise go.

If you don't know what's bothering you it's hard to work on it, and this may block you mentally and/or physically. Naming the problem will help get it out of the way. This exercise does not involve blaming yourself or others but rather becoming aware of the situations that put you on edge. These may include first readings of a script, working with a new director, and working with an actor who has a different style from your own. Once you understand the situations that make you uncomfortable, you might resist them less. And as you work on them, they will become easier.

PROCRASTINATION

- Sit comfortably.
- Without thinking through your Alexander directions, think about something you've been meaning to do but have put off.
- Think about a second and third thing you've been procrastinating about as well. Stay focused on those things.
- Attempt to put those things out of your mind. (Are you able to?)
- Notice how you're sitting.

We procrastinate all the time. It often feels harmless. People are often not aware that it's out of fear and anxiety. Often people grip their muscles and hold their breath when deciding whether to go to the gym or not. Experiment with thinking about things you may be conflicted about. Let your breath flow, and let your body be free as you do so.

FEAR

- Lie down on the floor, on your back. Make sure you are lying on an exercise mat, rug, or carpet.
- Place a softcover book or two under your head so that it's raised two to three inches off the floor.
- Bend your knees and place your feet on the floor.
- Put your hands on your lower rib cage.
- Think through your Alexander directions.
- Think of something that makes you a little bit afraid. Say you're running late for class. The bus or subway won't come, and you're stuck waiting, watching the minutes tick by. If you want to up the stakes, you can imagine you're running late for an audition. Stay with that thought.
- Notice what happens to your body and your breathing. You may sense some tightening.

- See if you can continue to think of what you're afraid of and not take the fear into your body.
- Let that thought go. Return to your Alexander directions and easy breath.

Notice I'm not going to tell you simply to not be afraid or to "just relax" in challenging circumstances. Giving yourself those direct instructions may not work. Similarly, willpower, or "the ability to control your own thoughts and behavior, especially in difficult situations" (according to the online *Cambridge Dictionary*), is not easy to exercise. And in attempting to strengthen their willpower, people often push, force, and tense up. There are softer ways to approach the problem of dealing with fear and resistance. Instead of trying hard, try soft.

BREAKING THINGS INTO UNITS

- Sit comfortably at a desk or table with a pen and paper, your laptop, or your phone.
- Choose an activity you find challenging or you tend to put off—going to the gym, for example, or buying fresh vegetables to cook.
- Think about the activity. Get a sense of why you are resisting it.
- Note what happens in your body as you think about it.
- Thinking through your Alexander directions, allow your breath to flow.
- Make a list of small units, or steps, involved in the activity. For example:

  1 Collect gym clothes.
  2 Put them in my gym bag.
  3 Find my car keys. (And so on.)

- Look at the first step on your list. Keep breathing. Stay easy in your neck and shoulders. Imagine yourself doing the first step.
- Repeat this for every step in the activity.

See if you can allow some of the resistance to melt away as you work through all the steps on your list. Breaking the activity into units will make it seem less overwhelming, and maintaining your poise throughout will make the activity feel more possible.

WHO IS MY RESISTANCE?

- Lie down on the floor, on your back. Make sure you are lying on an exercise mat, rug, or carpet.
- Place a softcover book or two under your head so that it's raised two to three inches off the floor.
- Bend your knees and place your feet on the floor.
- Put your hands on your lower rib cage.
- Think through your Alexander directions. Allow yourself to be quiet and easy.
- Go through the "voices in your head" that may say critical things to you.
- Stay as easy in your body as possible.
- Whom do these voices belong to?

Many people unconsciously internalize negative voices in their heads. They admonish themselves with thoughts such as "Do you really think you're going to get anywhere with acting?" Or "You know you're not that good, right? That other student always does better in class than you do." Or "You do so well when you're rehearsing in your room. Why can't you do as well in an audition?" These thoughts pull you out of focusing on what you're supposed to be doing—playing the scene. They can lead to resistance in a number of areas, physical and mental. They might represent what you're afraid your parents, teachers, or peers might be thinking. Or they may be completely imaginary. Rather than attempting to push them away, acknowledge they're there. Tell them you don't believe what they say and ask them to be quiet while you're working. Tell them you'll deal with them after class or after the performance but not *during* your performance. Later, when the class or performance is over, you can question the assumptions the voices are making.

PERFORMANCE ANXIETY

- Sit comfortably.
- Close your eyes and focus on your breathing.
- Imagine a performance situation in which you might get anxious: forgetting a line, being late for an entrance, being out of sync with the director.
- Try to stay with the feeling, yet simultaneously stay with your body and a free sense of breath.
- Whisper "ah" three times.
- Allow yourself to be slightly uncomfortable but still centered.
- Let the thought of anxiety go. Breathe out, release your body, and know the exercise is over.

It's common in performance for there to be moments when you step outside your comfort zone. Sometimes there is a tendency to pull away from these moments. But see if there is a way you can at least tolerate these moments, if not embrace them, and at the same time, in Alexander lingo, stay with yourself. Release your body as much as you can, let go of your breathing as much as possible, and find a way of being that works for you in the situation. During moments of stage fright, the mind jumps around and imagines worst-case scenarios. If you come back to yourself and focus on what you're doing, many of the fears will disappear. You can help yourself even more by finding a mantra that works for you, such as "I'll be okay," or "It will be all right," or "I'm prepared."

MAKING ROOM FOR WHO YOU ARE

- Lie down on the floor, on your back. Make sure you are lying on an exercise mat, rug, or carpet.
- Place a softcover book or two under your head so that it's raised two to three inches off the floor.
- Bend your knees and place your feet on the floor.
- Put your hands on your lower rib cage.

- Think through your Alexander directions.
- Let yourself feel like a hollow container.
- Allow yourself to be quiet for a few moments. Allow your whole body to be as free as possible.
- Have a sense of what it's like to be fully yourself, to allow for room for all your aspects in the hollow container that is your self. There's plenty of room for everyone.

On the page, this may look like a simple exercise. In practice, it may be one of the hardest exercises in the book. I'm not asking you to define all of who you are. I'm just asking you not to cut off parts of yourself. You are a wonderfully multifaceted human being with all kinds of different impulses. That's why you want to be an actor: to have a way to fully explore all colors. At this point in your development it's freeing to let yourself get a little messy—and surprise yourself a little. You'll be happy you did.

Primary Exercise

WORKING WITH RESISTANCE, NOT AGAINST IT

- Sit comfortably at a desk or table with a pen and paper, your laptop, or your phone.
- Think through your Alexander directions.
- Make a list of your important acting goals.
- Make a list of what you do well as an actor and what you may need to work on.
- Make a general timeline for working on these things.
- Review what you've written.
- Scan your body. What's happening with your head–neck relationship? What's happening with your shoulders and back? What's happening with your breathing?

- Stand and walk around the room letting yourself lengthen and widen.
- Come up onto your toes. Let your arms stretch out to either side.
- Return to your Alexander directions. See if you can review your lists with mind–body poise and free breathing.

Earlier in the chapter I asked you to think about things that make you a little bit afraid. But the things I'm asking you to think about here are much more emotionally charged. It won't be surprising if you catch yourself tensing muscles and making your breath shallow. But with practice you can think about challenging issues and still maintain a kind of equilibrium. This will benefit you in performing situations as well as in challenging life circumstances.

6 THE MIND–BODY CONNECTION

For loving, all my noblest, tenderest feelings are awakened,
And I become too great to be ashamed.
SUI SIN FAR, *THE BIRD OF LOVE*, 1910

One of the most important things for an actor to have is a strong mind–body connection. So much else flows from that. For example, you are born with talent, but it needs to be developed, and one of the best ways to develop it is to strengthen the mind–body connection. It's like a pipeline for your artistic impulses. You have the impulse, and your mind–body, as I call it, helps carry it out. If your mind–body is not fully attuned to your impulses, you may be unwittingly blocking some of your best work.

The National Institutes of Health defines mind–body medicine as focusing on:

- the interactions among the brain, the rest of the body, the mind, and behavior, and

- the ways in which emotional, mental, social, spiritual, experiential, and behavioral factors can directly affect health.

In other words, all parts of ourselves are connected—and this principle applies in the arts as well as in medicine. If you consciously encourage the mind–body connection, it will have a positive impact on all aspects of your functioning.

Emergence of the Mind–Body Concept

When F. M. Alexander developed his work, in the 1890s, the mind and the body were seen as separate. The mind was viewed as superior to the body. Now people feel differently. We all know that mental stress will affect your body and that physical stress will affect your mind and emotions. But we also know that as you calm and balance one part of your self, the other parts will also be positively affected. The Alexander Technique can be an important catalyst for this coordination of your whole self. It is a practical way that you can improve and strengthen your mind–body connection through working with awareness, inhibition, and direction.

Practical Application of the Mind–Body Concept

Remember the Sound Container exercise in Chapter 3 (page 47)? A partner traced you on a large piece of paper, then you used markers or crayons to fill in the places where your voice was vibrating. What you filled in and what you left out may have given you some clues about your own mind–body connection. You may have left out parts of yourself because they may not be at the forefront of your consciousness. This is not uncommon.

It's challenging to keep all aspects of yourself—mind, body, breath, voice, emotions—in your awareness and perfectly balanced at all times, but you can get better at remembering them as you practice. As you become more conscious of the connection and practice strengthening it, you'll train your mind and body to work together more constructively.

Applying the Mind–Body Concept to Acting

Teachers and directors often warn actors not to get stuck in their heads or overthink things. To me this means that they don't want actors to become overly self-conscious or inhibited by negative thoughts crowding their brains and impeding their creativity. This kind of *mental tension* affects the body, too, and leads to physical tension. It can also work the other way around. Anxiety or nerves can make actors tense their muscles, which will lead to greater mental and emotional tension. A tight body makes it harder to access the imagination and emotional life.

QUESTIONS FOR YOUR INNER SELF

1 What is your definition of the mind–body connection?
2 Do you tend to be "mind dominant" or "body dominant"?
3 How might the mind–body connection influence your acting?

It's useful to adopt what Alexander called a **correct mental attitude**, which may sound slightly Victorian and strict. But all it means is approaching things positively and with an open mind. It sounds easy enough. But when nerves, fear, and anxiety show up, correct mental attitude can go straight out the window. So remind yourself as often as you can of your commitment to it. Perhaps the most important thing is to remain *open to change*—specifically, to change within *yourself*. That means giving up the desire to be perfect all the time. It also means attempting not to end-gain (page 153). Experience shows that the more you focus on the *moment-to-moment* process, the better the result. By contrast, paradoxically, the more you focus on the result, the more your work seems forced or preplanned.

Tension and the Mind–Body Connection

It's my strong belief that you—and all actors—have unique creative impulses. Mental-physical tension can get in the way of these impulses. Taking away what you don't need—tension, tightness, restriction, and holding, both mental and physical—is vital. It will help you with your:

- **kinesthesia** ("awareness of the position and movement of the parts of the body by means of sensory organs [proprioceptors] in the muscles and joints," *English Oxford Living Dictionary*);

- **sensory awareness** ("the ability to receive and differentiate sensory stimuli," *Miller-Keane Encyclopedia and Dictionary of Medicine, Nursing, and Allied Health*);

- **consciousness** (a "set of ideas, attitudes, and beliefs," online *Collins Dictionary*);

- **emotions** ("strong feeling[s] deriving from one's circumstances, mood, or relationships with others," *Oxford English Dictionary*); and

- **intelligence** ("the ability to learn or understand or to deal with new or trying situations ... *also*: the skilled use of reason," online *Merriam-Webster Dictionary*).

The relieving of tension and stress in the mind and body, and in all aspects of the self mentioned above, will help strengthen your mind–body connection, which helps to improve your functioning in everyday life.

OPENNESS TO CHANGE

Openness to change can be difficult to achieve, but we want to do whatever we can to encourage it. A sense of safety has a lot to do with it, which is why strong personal boundaries when in a professional situation are always necessary. When you are doing a scene, find a way to feel safe enough within yourself, and within the room, for you to access your deepest creativity, to feel free enough to go wherever you need to go. One of the best ways to do this is by using the mind–body connection. That is, if you release the total self, your body and mind, you'll have a more direct connection to everything inside of you.

Being Present and the Mind–Body Connection

One of the most challenging aspects of the mind–body relationship may be the specter of time. Many of us have worries or regrets about the past.

In addition, we may have concerns or anxieties about the future. That makes it hard for us to be "in the moment," or "present," which is what many acting teachers say is one of the most important elements of good acting. So how do you stay in the present moment? One way is to not worry about the past—the past is gone. You can certainly learn from it, but you don't want to get stuck in it.

And just because you had a particular problem in the past doesn't mean that it has to repeat itself: you can change. Moreover, just as the past is out of our control, in a certain way so is the future. When you are in a play, for example, you prepare at home—you work on the character's objectives and motivations, you analyze the text, learn about the world of the play, learn your lines, work on the character's movement and speech. But when it comes time for opening night, you have to trust that you have done your homework. You have to let that work go. This will reduce your worry about what is about to happen in the immediate future and bring you into the present moment.

Sometimes being in the moment can be a little scary. You can be aware of your own concerns about measuring up, about doing everything right, about the audience liking you. I have a radical suggestion: put those concerns aside. They are legitimate concerns, but they won't help you on stage or on the set. You can think about them when the performance is finished. Instead, follow the simplest Alexander Technique advice: *keep breathing*. That is one of the best ways to foster a strong mind–body connection. Notice I didn't say, "Take a breath" or even "Breathe." Sometimes these instructions, though well meant, can lead people to suck in air or breathe in a tense way. The objective is to breathe as naturally and freely as possible, which gives you the inner freedom you need to act.

THE WHOLE SELF

There are many aspects of the self: mental, emotional, physical, intellectual, spiritual. But so often we're used to thinking of ourselves in pieces. Physical coordination certainly helps to bring things into alignment. You might also think of the mind–body connection as a silk thread that weaves itself through all your parts and helps tie them together. When you are fully living with the whole self, you experience more: you see more clearly, hear more acutely, and all your senses are heightened. Even more important for acting, you are far more able to listen to your acting partners while remaining available within yourself. The acting teacher Stella Adler put it vividly when she said that when you listen to your scene partner, "you must listen with your blood." This is an example of using your whole self in activity.

Process Versus Results

F. M. Alexander was very forward-thinking. He developed many process-oriented ways of working before these practices—which had been in place in Asia for centuries—became known elsewhere. He was Zen before the Western world really knew what that meant. In his time it was common to feel that "the end justifies the means." Many people still believe that today. There are situations where perhaps forcing and pushing for results can be effective, at least some of the time. But in acting for the stage and screen, this is often not the case. Tightness restricts the breathing, the voice, and movement. It stops the actor from being their most expressive. Alexander saw that if you pay attention to the process, all the small steps along the way, that this would indirectly give you a better result. With poise and balance, you will achieve a better result than with force. That's why I call Alexander Zen before his time.

The Alexander Process and Strengthening the Mind–Body Connection

Consider the example of breathing. The fact is that many of us, many times a day, make the breath shallow or sometimes hold the breath altogether. The first step is to recognize this through awareness. Your teachers and coaches may point it out to you, but you can give yourself a verbal cue when you catch yourself doing it. Thinking about it a few times a day can really make a difference. When you sense it, you can change it by asking yourself to stop your habit (inhibition) and do something new (direction).

What will happen in the future (the next moment) will blossom from the present (the current moment). Take a curious and exploratory stance: you don't have to know everything and get it right the first time—you can learn as you go. This constant learning will reinforce and strengthen a healthy mind–body connection.

GIVING YOURSELF TIME

The well-known Alexander teacher Walter Carrington was at one time an assistant to F. M. Alexander. Carrington used to say, "The greatest gift you can give yourself is time." There are many ways you can apply this to your own life. If you are cast in a play, for example, you can research the world of the play, read the script a number of times, and ponder the characters and their relationships far in advance of the first rehearsal. This is one way of giving yourself time.

Another way is to be patient with yourself when learning a new skill. Let's say you're a bit apprehensive about learning stage combat. If you give yourself time, however, you can avoid jumping to conclusions such as "I don't like stage combat, and I'm never going to be good at it." You can be patient with yourself in class as you slowly take in what the teacher is saying. You can give yourself time to practice at home. Gradually you will become more comfortable with stage combat. You might even come to like it.

Carrington was right: the biggest gift you can give yourself as an actor is the gift of time—the time to develop as an artist. Not just while you are in school but also in your professional career, over the course of your whole working life.

Writing, Trying Hard, and Trying Soft

When it comes to the mind–body connection, there is one activity that demonstrates its importance particularly well: writing. The words in your mind will never see the light of day unless you use your body—your hands and fingers—to help them get out. Perhaps this is why people's habits of writing, whether with a pen and paper or on a keyboard, are so strong.

Children learn how to write when they are very young and impressionable. In the process, it's common for them to grip their pens tightly to "get their letters right." Somehow we hold on to these habits into adulthood. As we grip the pen tightly, we tighten the neck, hunch the shoulders, squeeze the breath, and generally "try too hard." We do this in many other activities, too—going up and down stairs, bending, twisting and turning. The list is long.

On the other hand, if your intention is something like "try soft," change can happen. That is, if we clarify the mind–body connection and have a clear intention, there can be a different use of the self. The intention begins in your mind, then travels through your nervous system to your muscular system. You cue yourself to behave differently.

For example, if you decide not to give yourself a hard time but simply do your best in preparing a scene, then perform it to the best of your ability that day, you may be pleasantly surprised by the results. When you have a creative impulse—when you are not mentally or physically blocked—you can follow through on your instinct easily and freely, and it will feel like you are "in the zone."

Your Self, Inside and Out

With time and practice you will come to trust that using inhibition and direction will help bring you in tune with your mind–body connection. Rather than thinking of your body as it appears on the surface, you will think of it as it functions on the inside. For example, when you look in the mirror to check the appearance of your hair and clothing, you are looking at your body superficially. That's fine, and you want to look nice—but you also want to go deeper.

Find a website or an anatomy app that will give you a clear sense of how your spine is shaped and where it is in your body. Study the shape of the rib cage, the pelvis, the arms, and the legs. It's also helpful to look at the major muscles groups of the back, the abdomen, and so on. When you understand the way you are designed inside, you can move and function better.

Allowing yourself the awareness of the full volume of your physical self will bring you into a new relationship with your mental self. It's not possible to completely separate them. Being aware of this connection and working with it will bring the various aspects of your self in sync. This will affect you deeply in your life and in your performance.

JOURNAL

1   Write about the positive ways your mind works with your body during various physical activities, such as when you practice the Alexander Technique, yoga, or a dance routine.

2   Write down positive verbal cues you can use when you catch yourself admonishing yourself. For example, if you think, "I always freeze up when I have an emotional scene," you can write something like, "When an emotional scene is coming up, I'll let my breath flow and let my body be open and free. Then I'll be ready."

Exercises

TRYING HARD: WRITING

- Sit at your computer or sit at a table with a pen and paper.
- Write or type as you would normally.
- Notice your habits. Do you hold your breath? Do you hunch over the computer or paper? Do you tighten your fingers and wrists? What's happening with your arms? Your neck?
- Pause. Think through your Alexander directions.
- Try writing again, this time about something that is very important to you.
- Pause. Notice what's happening in your body and breath.
- Go back and forth between your habitual way of writing and the "Alexander way." What differences do you observe?

The way we write is so personal. We learn to do it at a young age, and our ways of doing it are ingrained, like our ways of speaking and walking: they seem fundamental to who we are. But it is possible to change *how* you write if you want to. For example, it's tempting to pull forward and down when you're writing or typing. But if you need to get closer to what you're doing, you can *lean forward from your hips.* You can open yourself across your chest and shoulders so you don't round yourself forward. This will help your breathing, and your back will be less tired if you are typing for a long period. These principles also apply when you're eating or having a cup of coffee. You don't need to pull down to reach your food or drink; you can bring the food or drink up to your mouth.

TRYING SOFT: PICKING UP OBJECTS

- Sit comfortably next to a table with some objects on it, including a book and a coffee cup.
- Think through your Alexander directions. Sit at your full height. Allow yourself to be long and wide.
- Remaining long and wide, pick up the book off the table.
- Keep breathing as you do so. Leave your hand, wrist, and arm easy.
- Replace the book on the table.
- Pick up the coffee cup as you leave yourself open and free.
- Stay easy and flowing in your body as you replace the coffee cup.
- Try this with other objects.

KEEP THE BREATH FLOWING

- Stand easily.
- Imagine you are tense or worried.
- Tune in to what you feel in your body. Where in your mind–body did you tighten up?
- Let that go. Think through your Alexander directions.

- Have the image of letting your breath flow in and out easily. Allow it—don't push it.
- Picture waves gently coming in and going out at the shore. Your breath can move in and out just as freely.

FINDING YOUR PERSONAL CENTER

- Sit comfortably at your computer, with your phone, or with your journal.
- Be aware of the way you're sitting and breathing.
- Think through your Alexander directions.
- Allow your breath to keep flowing.
- Without thinking about it too much, write a list of the things that make you feel good, safe, and taken care of.
- Review the list. Is there a common element to all or most of them?
- Return to thinking through your Alexander directions as you contemplate your list.

In a way, this is the opposite of the exercises in which I asked you to think about things that make you uncomfortable or fearful. What did you notice about your body and your breathing as you thought about the good things? Sometimes there is an easing in your psychophysical self— but at other times you will still feel somewhat locked in your body. As your sensory awareness becomes more acute, and you remind yourself about easy breathing and your Alexander directions, it can all begin to shift.

CALMING THE MIND AND THE BODY

- Sit comfortably.
- Think through your Alexander directions. Allow yourself to be at your full height and width. Let the breath be low and slow.
- Scan yourself for mental and physical tension.
- Use inhibition and direction to let your mind and body quiet themselves.

- Place your hands on top of your head, elbows to the side. This helps open the shoulders and chest.
- Place your hands around one of your knees, then bring it up toward your chest to ease your lower back.
- Gently lower your knee back to its original position.
- Repeat with the other knee.
- Whisper "ah" a few times (page 44).
- Let your mind and body be quiet.

Actors and acting students have demanding schedules. There are classes, homework, rehearsals, and getting to the gym when you can. That doesn't leave lots of time for centering. It helps to come to a "full stop" and open yourself to a different way of being. This exercise can be especially useful when preparing to go into an audition room.

THINKING YOUR WAY INTO YOUR BODY

- Stand comfortably.
- Think through your Alexander directions. Allow for flow through your body and your breath.
- Look at your right arm and hand.
- Think of your arm growing out of your back.
- Allow your arm to float straight out in front of you.
- Continue to think of your back lengthening and widening as you support your arm in space.
- See if you can stay with your mind, your Alexander directions, and your body at the same time.
- Float your arm back down.
- Repeat with your other arm. Then float both arms up at the same time.

LETTING GO OF OVERTHINKING

- Stand comfortably, with your feet a bit apart.
- Think through your Alexander directions.
- Have the image of your head being empty.

- Whisper "ah" three times (page 44).
- Allow your head to curve over toward your chest.
- Slowly let your whole body round over toward the floor until you are hanging all the way over, with your knees bent.
- Allow your arms to hang toward the floor. Let your neck and shoulders be very free. Nod your head a few times to make sure you're not holding on.
- Slowly unroll up. Initiate the movement from your core. Build up your spine one vertebra at a time. Your neck and head are the last things to come up.
- Whisper "ah" three more times. Imagine your head is empty or full of helium.

Getting "stuck in your head" can be one of the main problems of acting. Rather than focusing on the character you're playing, you end up worrying about what the other actors think of you, whether the director likes you, and so on. When you're in this state, you are not actually doing your job, which is to be the character to the best of your ability that day. But if you can take yourself out of your head—i.e., stop judging what you are doing as you are doing it—it can give you tremendous freedom.

MENTAL ATTITUDE

- Sit comfortably with a piece of paper and a pen, your laptop, or your phone.
- Make a list of physical tensions you are aware of in your body.
- Make a list of breathing tensions you're aware of.
- Make a list of mental attitudes you have that may get in the way of your acting.
- Pause and put the list down.
- Whisper "ah" a couple of times (page 44).
- Allow yourself to sit quietly for a minute or two.

Having negative beliefs about yourself or your abilities often ends up manifesting itself as tension in your body. It's ironic, because many of these unconstructive thoughts may be trying to "help" you. "Don't mess up." "You made that mistake again!" "Just talk fast and get it over with!" These kind of thoughts pull you out of a constructive mind–body relationship and away from your character's objectives. Once you become aware of your unconstructive mental habits and understand them better, you can catch yourself before you get into them again. And you can gently nudge yourself toward a new way of being.

THINKING IN ACTIVITY

- Sit comfortably.
- Think through your Alexander directions.
- Letting yourself remain mentally and physically poised, stand up out of the chair.
- Think through your Alexander directions again.
- Walk across the room.
- Think through your Alexander directions again.
- Pick something up.
- Go through all the actions again as you think through your directions.

Many people say, "I can't think about more than one thing at a time." And yet people, especially performers, do this all the time. Consider opera singers, for example. As they perform, they are dealing with music, lyrics, an unfamiliar language, movement, acting, and watching the conductor all at the same time. So certainly you can think about inhibition and direction as you go about your activities.

It's easiest in the beginning to apply the principles when the activity is simple: brushing your teeth, putting on your shoes, standing waiting for a light to change, sitting and reading. Because these activities don't require much complex thought, you can take stock (use your awareness), inhibit ("I don't want to slump while I'm reading"), and direct ("Let my neck be free, to let my head go forward and up, to let my torso lengthen and widen, to let my arms and legs release away from my body so I can sit at my full height as I read"). You can continue whatever activity you're engaged in as you make a change in yourself. Or you can take a split second to pause, then make the change. Someone watching you wouldn't know what you're doing—it wouldn't be apparent.

Another example of thinking in activity is when I walk through Grand Central Station or Times Square during rush hour. There are enormous numbers of people walking in all kinds of directions. You can feel them rushing, and some of them are quite tense. I don't want to imitate that rushing and tension, so I think in activity. As I walk, I remind myself to lengthen and widen so I don't hunker down and lean forward to barrel through the crowd. I also remind myself to let my breath keep flowing. This gives me a much more pleasant experience.

FLOW

- Stand comfortably at your full height.
- Think through your Alexander directions.
- Walk forward.
- Walk backward.
- Return to your starting position.
- Turn and walk to your left.
- Turn and walk to your right.
- Walk in a large circle. Then a small one.
- Walk in a figure eight.
- Walk, frequently changing directions.

People often think in short bursts, which results in movement that is somewhat jerky and tight. One of the main purposes of this exercise is to experiment with swift changes in direction that don't involve tension or jerky motions. The exercise helps create a "big picture" view of activity, so you can see how one thing leads to the next in an easy progression. This results in flowing motions.

UNPLUGGING

- Turn off your phone, your computer, and all devices—don't just silence them.
- Lie down on the floor, on your back. Make sure you are lying on an exercise mat, rug, or carpet.
- Place a softcover book or two under your head so that it's raised two to three inches off the floor.
- Bend your knees and place your feet on the floor.
- Put your hands on your lower rib cage.

- Scan yourself for tension.
- Think through your Alexander directions.
- Softly focus on your breath flowing in and out.
- Allow your body to gently melt toward the floor.
- Sense the support that comes from the floor.
- Let your mind be quiet.
- Give yourself time to do nothing but be with yourself—your mind–body.
- Allow your breath to flow gently in and out.

Turning off your devices signals that you are putting aside time to recharge. You will sense this at some deep level. People sometimes feel guilty taking time for themselves. But if your body becomes overtired, your productivity goes down and you're apt to make mistakes. So this exercise is not only restorative but also preventive.

Primary Exercise

ALIGNING THE MIND AND BODY

- Stand with your feet slightly apart.
- Scan yourself for mental and physical tension (awareness).
- Remind yourself you don't want to hold on (inhibition).
- Think through your Alexander directions (direction).
- Whisper "ah" twice (page 44).
- Allow your mind to be quiet.
- Stretch your arms out to either side. Release them down. Repeat.
- Stretch your arms up to the ceiling. Release them down. Repeat.
- Continue lengthening and widening as you walk forward five steps.
- Walk backward to your original position.
- Whisper "ah" again as you move your arms around in a large circle.
- Once again, allow your mind to be quiet.

In everyday life there are so many things we have to *accomplish*. Sometimes it can seem like life is nothing more than one long to-do list. It's rare that we give ourselves the opportunity to step out of our daily routines and "return to the self." This exercise will only take a few minutes, but if you give yourself over to it and temporarily put aside all the things you need to do, it will refresh you, just as one might refresh a web page on a computer. You can return to neutral and start anew after practicing it.

7 CLASSES AND REHEARSALS

Be yourself. Everyone else is taken.

ATTRIBUTED TO OSCAR WILDE

I dwell in possibility.

EMILY DICKINSON

At this point, you've learned about the three vital components of the Alexander Technique: awareness, inhibition, and direction. We've covered how these components can be applied to the building blocks of your acting: balance, coordination, movement, breath, and voice. But how do you work on these building blocks, not in isolation but as an organic part of everything you're studying in the drama department?

Classes

The first place you can apply what you've learned is in class, because it's easier to change your mind–body habits in a class situation than it is in rehearsal, where the stakes are higher. For example, in addition to acting and scene study, you may be taking classes in voice, speech, dance, singing, and other subjects, including theater history. Following are some of the activities the Alexander Technique can help you with in any of those classes:

- Sitting
- Observing
- Listening

- Responding and talking
- Taking the leap

You might look at the list above and think that you already know how to do everything. I'm sure you do. But the Alexander principles will help you accomplish each of these tasks more simply, efficiently, and easily.

Sitting

Everyone knows how to sit, even infants. And yet it's one of the activities that students complain about the most. You have to sit many hours a day— in class, in the library, in rehearsals, and at home at the computer. But although how *long* you sit may be out of your control, the *way* you sit is definitely under your control. I advise you to review the discussion of the mechanics of sitting on page 70. In addition, there are ways to counteract the effects of uncomfortable chairs, some of which may be too high, too low, or too deep. There is no one chair that is perfect for every body type.

Some of the worst kinds of chairs used in colleges and universities are the familiar inexpensive metal and plastic folding chairs. The metal chairs often lean back at an awkward angle, and the seat is somewhat curved. This leads to people slumping uncomfortably, usually after only a few minutes. The thin plastic chairs tend not to give much support and are often designed with an unsupportive back. This also encourages people to slump down.

Occasionally an institution will buy a limited number of expensive "ergonomically designed chairs." But you can sit inefficiently in any kind of chair. Even an ostensibly well-designed chair that doesn't fit your body can be challenging to sit in. *You need to be aware of how you are using yourself in the chair to avoid pain and strain.*

STRATEGIES FOR UNCOMFORTABLE CHAIRS

In a classroom, you don't have a choice as to what you sit on. You need to do the best you can with what you have. So take a few minutes to examine the chairs in your room.

- Analyze the height as it relates to your height.

- Analyze the depth of the seat as it relates to the length of your legs.
- Get a sense of what kind of support (or lack thereof) the back of the chair gives.
- What is the angle of the back relative to the seat?

Then come up with strategies for being as balanced and supported as possible, even in a less-than-perfect chair. Make sure to be sitting directly on top of your sitting bones.

- If the chair is too low for you, try sitting on some books or blankets to bring yourself up a little higher.
- If it's too high, try propping your feet on something or sitting forward toward the front edge of the chair.
- Try putting something behind your lower back—a rolled up sweater, for example—to help you stay lengthened and widened.
- Sitting forward can also be helpful if the chair is too deep or in some way encourages you to slump. This also works if the chair seat tips you too far back.
- When sitting forward toward the edge of the chair, you will be most supported if you have your feet flat against the floor.

If you lengthen and widen, the core muscles in your midriff will help support you. If your back gets tired when you're sitting forward in the chair, you can rest against the back of the chair for short periods. *If you have a good chair seat and back, it's fine to sit at the back of the chair. Be at your full height and width as you do so.*

This way of sitting—maintaining optimal use by releasing up into length and out into width while allowing your breath to flow—is what I call **active sitting**. It is a *natural* way to sit. Slumping down, on the other hand, is a *habitual* way of sitting. It's hard on the body and difficult to sustain for hours at a time. It also tends to restrict breathing.

Observing

Observing is one of the most important things you will do in your classes. Of course you will learn a great deal when you get up to perform monologues and scenes. But you may learn even more by observing your teacher and fellow students.

Watch their body language. How do they use their bodies? What kind of coordination do you see? How does this affect their movement and gestures? What do you notice about the physicality of the actors as they interact in a scene? Does that physicality mostly suit the characters they are playing? Are there certain things the actors could work on to even more fully embody their roles? What are your general impressions of the characters and the play itself?

As you observe, it's ideal to be in an open, receptive state. That means being nonjudgmental and supportive. It can be stressful for student actors to get up in front of a class and play a scene. You want to be sympathetic to that, and you'd like your fellow actors to be supportive of you when it's your turn.

On the other hand, *you don't want to absorb other people's tension.* If you can see the actors struggling with nerves, don't assume their burden. Leave yourself free in your body and breathing. It's easy to fall into the habit of tightening your body if you see someone else doing it. That goes for when you're playing a scene, too. Don't let yourself imitate your acting partner's tension.

Listening

We think we know how to listen. But often our minds wander, and the next thing we know we're thinking about things not happening in the room. *One way to check if you are listening is if your eyes are glazed.* If they are, even slightly, you're not fully hearing everything that's being said. Really listening requires being in your body. You listen with your ears, your sense of hearing, of course, but at the highest level, you can listen with almost a sixth sense.

In this way listening can meld with your visual sense, your observation. You can pick up an enormous amount of information even over a short period of time if you listen with your eyes as well as your ears. You can listen to *what* is being said, *how* it's being said, and what is *not* being said. This applies when your fellow actors are playing a scene as well as when there is a classroom discussion.

It's common for acting teachers to suggest that actors listen to what's going on in a scene as if they're hearing it for the first time. You, the actor, have read and memorized the dialogue, but your character has never heard it before. I saw this demonstrated to an extraordinary degree when I saw Judi Dench on stage in *Amy's View*. Much of the time she was quite still, yet alert. She seemed to drink in every word the other actors said. I've never seen such a clear example of "hearing for the first time." There was no tension in her body at all. No barrier between her and the other actors. I also did not see her "prepare" to say her next line. It simply came out of her, completely organically.

If you are tight in your body, it is challenging for you to fully listen. When you are stiff, it's almost as if you are pulled out of what is happening in the room and locked inside yourself. Even if the tenor of the room seems somewhat hostile, there is no reason for you to tense up, too. Returning to your directions will help you stay as free as possible. Keeping your breath flowing, low and slow—especially if you are nervous or uncertain of the environment—will also help. You want to stay on an even keel as you listen to and participate in class discussions. This will help you be *in the moment*—the state every actor seeks to achieve.

Responding and Talking

When you're listening, you take in a great deal of information. Once you take in that information, you have an impulse. And if you choose to act on that impulse, you respond, either verbally or nonverbally.

A nonverbal response can be anything from a facial expression to a slight movement of your body to a series of jumping jacks. It could also involve doing nothing but sitting stock-still. It depends on the situation and the context. A verbal response could be anything from saying a line as written to paraphrasing it (if you're doing that as an exercise) to improvising. A verbal response is sometimes accompanied by physical behavior, too, of course.

Whatever type of response you have, it will be blocked or altered if tension gets in the way. On one end of the tension spectrum is preplanning your response; on the other end is wildly and erratically overreacting, neither of which is ideal. Both of these extremes can be avoided by allowing yourself a degree of mental-emotional-physical freedom.

Reminding yourself before the scene begins of what your character wants can be a big help. So can going through your Alexander directions. But once you're in the scene, you're in it. You can't evaluate or judge yourself *as you are performing* because that means you're not really in the scene and are standing outside yourself in an unhelpful way.

Taking the Leap

"Taking the leap" is the phrase I would use to describe trust. Specifically, trusting yourself. I don't have to tell you that this is sometimes challenging to do. There are so many situations in which an actor can feel slightly, or not so slightly, insecure: you've just learned the scene, you don't know the other actors well, you've never worked with the director, it's a different kind of role from the ones you're used to playing—the list of possibilities is endless.

If you're feeling insecure, chances are you're thinking about worst-case scenarios rather than the character you're playing and the circumstances they're in. Yet *in spite of your insecurity, you need to take the leap into playing the character and the scene.*

How can you do that, practically? Research on stage fright shows that releasing your body and connecting to your breath are the best things you can do under these circumstances. Even if your nerves are only slightly frayed, it helps to come back to your Alexander directions—come back to your body. Allow your breath to be low and slow. This is a vital part of the process in class, in auditions, or in performance.

Rehearsals

Ideally, the classroom is a place to experiment, to try things out in a supportive environment. You learn a lot about yourself in class, including how you approach various kinds of material and how you work with other actors.

Rehearsals are different. The focus shifts from exploratory work to an end product: a production. It might be a workshop in a small theater or a large mainstage production. Regardless, you are a part of a team: actors, the director, the stage manager, and the design and production staff. There's lots to navigate!

There's one thing I can guarantee: everyone appreciates an actor who is prepared. As soon as possible, read the play. Read it as many times as you can before the first rehearsal. Research the playwright and their world, and research the world of the play. Make sure you learn your lines and are off book by the date the director requests it. All these things will help give you confidence in what you're doing and will reduce your stress level.

In addition, part of your homework is keeping yourself physically coordinated and balanced. This goes for your breathing as well. Whenever you can, warm up before class. Use the exercises in this book to help you get in touch with your body. You want to be free as possible physically so that you are open to the work at hand. You want the breath to be flowing easily. Any holding of the breath or shallow breathing will accumulate tension in your body.

Follow professional theater etiquette during rehearsal, which can be boiled down to:

- Always be on time. Better yet, be fifteen minutes early.
- Be friendly, flexible, and professional.
- Be supportive and constructive.

In addition, actors should follow a good self-care program to keep their stress levels at a minimum:

- Get plenty of sleep.
- Stay hydrated.
- Eat healthful food regularly.
- Exercise regularly.
- Practice the Alexander Technique.

Everything I said above about sitting, observing, listening, responding, talking, and taking the leap applies to rehearsals as well. But because the stakes are higher here, you may sense your body tightening a bit more.

Remind yourself briefly, whenever you can, to stay free in your body. Of course, most of your focus will be on what's happening in the rehearsal, but there will be moments when you can take time to "touch base":

- On the way to rehearsal.
- As you sit and wait for rehearsal to begin.
- During breaks.
- When you go to the restroom.
- When the director takes time to speak to the production team.

Even if your reminders are very short—a few seconds—they will make a difference. Instead of checking messages on your phone, turn these moments into opportunities for recharging yourself. Anytime we break a tension habit, it paves the way for new, more constructive ways of being. You are reprogramming your mind–body in constructive ways.

A Word about Auditions

Whether auditioning for a school play or a professional production, actors tend to get nervous. It's understandable. It feels like there is a lot at stake. Sometimes it feels personal, like you are being judged as a person. You've probably heard your teachers say this is not the case. Actors are evaluated in terms of their appropriateness for a role. Therefore, the more you can keep your focus on what you can control—your work—the better. This is the job of the actor.

If you can go through the Constructive Rest exercise (page 22) at home before you leave for the audition, that's ideal. In addition, I recommend:

- Getting seven or eight hours of sleep two nights before as well as the night before the audition.

- Working on your Alexander Technique the morning of the audition.

- Eating well and hydrating starting two days before the audition.

- Planning your wardrobe the night before. Lay out your clothes and everything else you need so they're easily accessible.

- Giving yourself plenty of time to get to the audition.

- Arriving early.

- Finding a quiet corner to prepare. You can be polite and say hello to other actors, but avoid socializing. You can always socialize after the audition.

JOURNAL

1   Make a note of the things that make you uncomfortable about classwork, rehearsals, and auditions. How do they manifest themselves in your body?

2　Write down the things you like about classwork, rehearsals, and auditions. Do you notice any good things happening in your body and breathing when you are comfortable in these situations?

3　In class or rehearsal, note how others are using their bodies in playing scenes. Write down tension habits you observe that you would like to avoid. Then list things you see in others' bodies and movement that you think are positive and would like to have yourself. Can you observe others objectively and nonjudgmentally?

Exercises

OBSERVING AND RESPONDING

- Stand with a partner. One of you has a bean bag.
- Toss the bean bag lightly and easily between you.
- Move a little bit apart as you continue to throw it.
- Move farther apart. Throw both underhand and overhand.
- Move around the room—closer and farther away from each other. Explore throwing the bag high and low, fast and slow, and in various patterns.

During this exercise, you will get into a rhythm with your partner. You'll go with what's happening, with the flow. You'll have a sense of what your partner is doing, and you'll respond accordingly. And you'll do it rather quickly, or you'll drop the bean bag. If you do, that's okay, of course, but you'll find that the easier you are in your body and breath, the easier the exercise.

NOT ANTICIPATING

- Find a partner to work with.
- Choose a scene you'll both work on.

- Think through your Alexander directions.
- Read the scene out loud.
- Focus on really listening to your partner when they are reading.
- Keep your breath flowing as your partner reads.
- Don't anticipate when it's "your turn."
- Don't hold your breath right before speaking your line. Let your breath naturally lead into speaking.

This is an exercise in listening and responding. Staying present, you'll be able to listen more fully and authentically. Making sure that your breath keeps flowing will help. Unconsciously, people often subtly brace the body before speaking. The moment right before you speak is called the **vocal onset**. Make sure that you don't hold your breath or squeeze it just at that moment. This is also a good moment to make sure you don't tighten your neck, pull your head back and down, and tighten your shoulders and back muscles.

STAYING PRESENT

- Sit comfortably at your full height, right on top of your sitting bones.
- Think through your Alexander directions.
- Let your breath flow.
- Be aware of the room—the space above, behind, and to either side of you.
- Be aware of everything that's happening in the room while still "staying with yourself."
- See if you can be aware of the external environment and your inner self at the same time. If not at the same time, you can go back and forth in your awareness from one to the other.

Being present is one of the most important skills an actor can have. It's a skill you can work on over a long period of time. It means being aware of the self and the outer world in a "three-dimensional" way. It also means not being pulled into too much concern about the past or the future. You consciously make the decision to be in the present moment. If you feel yourself pulling out of the moment (it happens), gently bring yourself back. You may need to do this a number of times. It's okay. The more you work on it, the better you will get at it.

PREREHEARSAL WARM-UP

- Get to your rehearsal early, before others arrive, or use a space near the rehearsal room. Giving yourself ten minutes to warm up before a rehearsal is ideal. If time is short, five minutes is still helpful.
- Take ten to fifteen minutes to go through the Constructive Rest exercise (page 22). If there isn't time, do it for five minutes.
- Remind yourself of your Alexander directions. Apply them to each part of your body, from head to toe.
- Go through the Blowing Out Air exercise (page 43).
- Go through the Whispered "Ah" exercise (page 44).
- Spend a few minutes sitting in a chair, thinking through your Alexander directions, opening yourself physically and in your breath, and allowing yourself to be ready for the work.

POSTREHEARSAL COOL-DOWN

- Stand with your feet a bit apart.
- Think through your Alexander directions.
- Walk around the room. Speed up and slow down. Whisper "ah" several times (page 44).
- Stop walking.
- Jump up and down several times, sighing as you do.
- Come to stillness.
- Slowly roll down through your spine. Let your head come toward your chest, and slowly roll over vertebra by vertebra until you are hanging all the way over (page 103).
- Whisper "ah" a few more times.
- Roll up, starting from your core, vertebra by vertebra. The last thing to come up is the neck, then the head.
- Gently turn your head from side to side a few times. Nod up and down a few times.
- Go through the Constructive Rest exercise (page 22) if you choose.

It's a good idea to give yourself a cool-down after rehearsal to help you transition back into everyday life. This is especially important if you are participating in long rehearsals or if the material you are working on is intense. You don't want to take the tension of the character and the play back home with you. You want to leave it in the rehearsal room.

SPLIT-SECOND PREPARATION

- Sit comfortably in class or rehearsal.
- Think through your Alexander directions. Let your breath flow.
- Make sure you're fully present and watching your colleagues work rather than being lost in your own world.
- When it is your turn to get up and do a scene, take a split second to let go of your whole body.
- Breathe out as you stand up.
- Exhale quietly as you walk to the place where you will do your scene.

The moment before beginning is a moment when people sometimes clutch and tighten. It's ironic, because that is the moment when we most need to let go. This exercise will help you ground yourself and stay in the present moment.

GIVING YOURSELF A MANTRA

- Sit or lie down comfortably.
- Think through your Alexander directions. Allow yourself to come into a quiet, focused place.
- Imagine you are about to do a scene in class, in a rehearsal, or at an audition.
- Rethink your Alexander directions to help you stay easy and connected to your body.
- Let your breath be low and slow.
- Find a simple mantra for yourself along the lines of "I'm ready," "I'm prepared," or "I'm ready to go."

Research shows that positive self-talk can make a big difference when we're trying to reduce tension. Nerves can lead us into catastrophizing—imagining complete and utter failure. That doesn't mean you have to go to the other extreme and tell yourself you're going to give the best performance in history. But simple, calm reminders that you have rehearsed and prepared, and that you know what you're doing, seem to do the trick. Right before doing a scene is not the moment to become self-judgmental and self-conscious. Leave the analysis for another time. Now is the time to quietly focus on what you're about to do.

PERMISSION TO PLAY

- Sit comfortably in class or in rehearsal.
- Allow yourself to be at your full height and width.
- Let your breath be easy.
- Imagine that your head is hollow.
- Imagine that your whole body is hollow.
- Let your whole body be light and easy.
- Give yourself permission to "play"—to give yourself to the rehearsal process, to let yourself tap into your boldest creative impulses.
- Remember your mantra. Then go.

HALLWAY WARM-UP

- Put your belongings somewhere safe and out of the way.
- Stand comfortably.
- Have a quick thought of being at your full height and open through your chest and shoulders.
- Place one hand over your mouth, as if you're yawning.
- Whisper "ah" (page 44) twice into your hand.
- Let your neck, shoulders, and back release as you breathe out.
- Remember your mantra.

You can practice this exercise as you wait outside the audition-room door. You can stand there casually, holding up your hand to your mouth as if you're yawning or thinking. That way no one will see that you are breathing out on a silent whispered "ah." This helps release you right before you go into the room.

ENTERING THE AUDITION ROOM

- Find a partner to work with.
- Ask your partner to play the part of a person holding an audition.
- Find a room to serve as the audition room. Stand outside the closed door.
- Take yourself through the Hallway Warm-Up exercise (page 121).
- Ask your partner to open the door.
- Exhale as you walk into the room.
- Bring a touch of the character you will be auditioning for into the room.
- Stand in the center of the room and smile.
- Keep your breathing easy.
- Say "Hi," and tell your partner your name if it was not announced.
- Exhale.
- Begin the scene or monologue.

Many teachers and acting professionals recommend that you enter an audition room "confidently." This exercise will help you release, which in turn gives you confidence. You don't need to enter as your character 100 percent, but you can bring a flavor of the character with you as you walk in. This allows the auditioners to see the character in you before you even begin to speak.

LEAVING THE AUDITION ROOM

- Stand easily, at your full height.
- Let your body be free and allow your breathing to be easy.

- Smile and say, "Thank you."
- Pick up your things quickly and efficiently, without rushing.
- Walk out of the room.

Believe it or not, this is a helpful exercise to practice. Many actors bring too many objects with them into the room. Then they struggle awkwardly, picking up assorted bags and attempting to banter wittily on their way out. You can follow the lead of the people leading the audition—if they want to chat, by all means chat! But if they signal silently that they want to move on to the next person, then it's part of your job to efficiently and gracefully leave the room. Make sure not to apologize after your audition. Allow your body to take up its full space as you leave. This will help give you presence.

Primary Exercise

PRIVATE WARM-UP

- Put your belongings somewhere safe and out of the way.
- Stand with your feet in a fairly wide stance.
- Sense the floor and the space between the top of your head and your feet.
- Think up and out through your body.
- Be aware of the front, back, and sides of you.
- Sense the space around you.
- Sigh twice.
- Whisper "ah" (page 44) twice.
- Stretch your arms out to the sides twice.
- Stretch your arms up toward the ceiling twice. The second time, come up onto your toes.
- Remember your mantra.

You can do this quick warm-up in the privacy of a bathroom stall or in an empty room before you go into an audition. It only takes one to three minutes, but it will help you "take the leap."

8 PERFORMANCE

I have come
from pride
all the way up to humility.

AMY LOWELL, "DAWNS"

This is everything you have been working for: performance. This is why you've enrolled in school, taken classes, prepared scenes and monologues, auditioned, and rehearsed. This is the culmination of your dream. And often it's a combination of intoxicating and terrifying. Every performer at one time or another is afraid of being judged: by the audience, the director, and their peers. But concern about what people think of you and your performance can sometimes lead to crippling worry and nerves. It's part of your job not to focus on being judged. *It's your job to play the part to the best of your ability today.*

But so many concerns can crowd your mind right before performing:

- What if I forget my lines?

- What if I don't know what I'm doing in this play?

- Maybe I'm completely wrong for this part.

- Maybe it was a mistake taking a role in this play; maybe I should have auditioned for the musical instead.

- What if I'm a fraud? And don't know how to act at all?

Anxiety and Performance

You'd be surprised how many actors, including well-known ones, have thoughts like these running through their heads. It's never comfortable, but it is especially unhelpful right before a performance. It distracts you from doing your job: acting.

Worry and anxiety are primary causes of being "in your head." This pulls you out of your body and out of the moment. It makes you less spontaneous and present. But one of the main benefits of the Alexander Technique is that it provides a pragmatic way for you to come into your body, stay connected to your breathing, and act on your creative impulses. All you have to do is use the tools you've practiced in lower-stakes situations and apply them to performance. Just because there is an audience observing you doesn't mean that you need to vocally or physically push. *Even though the situations are different, your job is the same. It's Sanford Meisner's famous definition of acting: "Living truthfully under imaginary circumstances."*

The Character's Physical Reality

An important part of following Meisner's invaluable advice is *investigating, exploring, and embodying your character's physical reality.* Each of us moves and behaves in a certain way as a result of certain factors outside our control. You are born into a family in a certain area of the country and are surrounded by a certain community. Just as you are affected by these things, so is your character. For example, people tend to imitate their family's movement and physicality. So it bears thinking about the physical lives of your character's family and community. Also, your character's profession and hobbies have an important effect on the way they move. If your character grew up on a farm in the early nineteenth century and spent most of the day engaged in activities such as tilling the land, lifting bales of hay, and riding horses, this would have a profound effect on their physical life. Thinking about all this will help you find a nuanced and detailed physicality, which in turn will aid you in embodying what seems to be a real person.

Another big part of the actor's job, I believe, is developing *presence and poise.* This will help you in everything you do, whether rehearsal or performance. Actors need to be quick-witted. Rehearsal time may be short; new scripts often go through many changes; the director may want to try things out. To be your best throughout the rehearsal and production process, ideally you want to be flexible, elastic, open, and embracing. Poise and presence will help you accomplish that. That way, when the unexpected happens—and it will—you'll be able to handle it gracefully. You can find presence and poise by releasing your body and your breath. First it's a matter of setting your intention, then working on it a little bit every day.

Preparation and Performance

You may have heard some of your teachers talk about how important preparation is. The more you prepare, the less likely it is that your nerves will rear their ugly heads. The more familiar you are with the material, the more you can free yourself in performance. Of course, rehearsal is a large part of your preparation. But in film, television, and video, you are expected to come with your lines memorized and ready to perform. A big part of preparation is what you do at home. Preparation is partly mental, partly emotional, and partly physical. By opening yourself up in all these areas, you will bring your best self to the work.

THE DIFFERENCES BETWEEN REHEARSING AND PERFORMING

The differences between rehearsing and performing might seem obvious. But your job in each is slightly different. Each director might handle things in a unique way, but usually in rehearsal you are becoming familiar with your character, the world of the play, and your acting and production colleagues. Under the best rehearsal circumstances you are allowed to explore and try things out. You're questioning and learning. Sometimes it's wise not to jump to conclusions quickly but rather allow things to evolve. Then, when it's performance time, all the rehearsing and home preparation somehow come together into an organic whole. Your task is to *allow* it to happen—not to present your performance in a neat little box but to live your character's reality as if for the first time. There are technical demands: the audience needs to hear you, there is blocking you need to follow, and so on. But even more important, in a best-case scenario, all your rehearsal and preparation will feed you as you live your character's truth. The Alexander Technique can assist by helping you be aware, flexible, and coordinated through both processes.

Physical Preparation

It's tempting when you get a script to dive right in. But I suggest you take a few minutes to lay the mental and physical groundwork first, before you read a scene out loud. Some actors prefer to do so in a perfectly quiet, dark room with no distractions. Others might like a bright, airy room with music or TV playing in the background. Still others prefer to have people around. It's important to find what works for you.

Once you've determined your ideal working environment, put aside a block of time for preparation. Some actors like to work in short segments; others prefer long stretches or alternating between short and long. But even if you are working in short segments of fifteen minutes each, it is worthwhile spending a minute or two bringing yourself into a calmly focused place by practicing some of the exercises in this book. Then you will have fertile ground on which to build.

As you become more practiced in opening your body, breath, and voice, you'll be able to bring yourself to center in a few minutes. This is a skill that will come in very handy in the professional acting world. Work on film sets sometimes is slow. You wait for a very long time to perform your scene. Then you are suddenly told that you'll be performing in a few minutes. You can use those valuable minutes to help bring yourself into your most creative place.

Mental Preparation

Mental preparation is perhaps even more important than physical preparation. Your mental way of being will profoundly affect what is happening in your body and your breath. In my experience, these are some of the most important ways to mentally prepare for a performance:

- Achieve clarity about who your character is and how the character is involved in the story being told. These ideas will have come from your work with the director and your teachers. What are the character's intentions? What are the obstacles? What is the character's arc in the story?

- Organize yourself. This means having everything you need laid out in advance in your bag, knowing your way to the theater, leaving yourself extra time so you won't be late, and staying on top of all the other mechanical details you have to deal with.

- Find a quiet, still center within yourself, even if your character is loud and frantic. You, the actor, will be able to play that character more effectively if you are mentally balanced.

MENTAL INTENTION

Peggy Ashcroft was a well-known English actor who worked in the early to mid-twentieth century. Her career spanned more than sixty years. In 1935 she played Juliet in what became a famous production of *Romeo and Juliet*. The renowned actors Laurence Olivier and John Gielgud played Romeo and Mercutio respectively; five weeks later, they switched roles, and Gielgud played Romeo to Olivier's Mercutio. Before the production opened, Ashcroft was noted for her acting as opposed to her appearance: she was not thought of as a stunning beauty. But it was widely noted how beautiful she looked in this particular role. A friend asked her how she achieved the effect. Ashcroft told her that every night she stood in the wings of the theater before she made her entrance and convinced herself that she was the most beautiful woman in the world. The audience definitely saw the effect of her mental preparation. This is one of my favorite acting stories. It shows how the power and clarity of thought can help the actor transform from within. Ashcroft did not use special makeup or wigs to change the way she looked. She used her internal experience to change her external appearance.

The Expansive Self

Standing on a stage, large or small, is an act of bravery. You are putting yourself on the line. People are looking at you: your body, your voice—they are listening to you speak, watching you move, and watching you experience the life of the character. This can make you feel vulnerable. But whereas a painter may feel vulnerable when their art is shown, they are physically separate from the art itself. An actor and their art, on the other hand, are in the same container. Art happens in the moment, in real time. It's one of the things that makes live theater and film unique. But it also presents challenges for the performer.

How can you play a vulnerable character without making yourself physically smaller? Or, conversely, how do you take up your full psychic space without coming across as cocky or overly confident? Part of it has to do with the space you're performing in: is it large or small, with good acoustics or echoing, casual or ornate and formal? In any of these different kinds of theaters, you can be your expansive self. It's always a good idea to spend as much time on the stage as possible before rehearsals. Walk around it, both as yourself and as your character.

Consider these questions:

- What is the stage like? How wide and deep is it? How high up is the ceiling?

- What is the shape of the stage? Is it a proscenium? Is it round?

- How big is the theater? How many seats are there? Is it wide or narrow?

- How far is the audience from the stage?

- What is the floor like underneath your feet? Does it make a noise?

- How many steps does it take to get from one side of the stage to the other? From downstage to upstage?

These spatial variables will affect everything you do with your body and voice.

THEATER SPACES

Chances are you will act in all kinds of performance spaces—some traditional, others not. You might perform a workshop production of a play in a classroom setting. That has a certain set of parameters. You're often very close to the audience. Because there is rarely professional lighting in this kind of space, you may see the audience. Make sure you don't pull away from them or make yourself smaller. Even when performing in a small room, you want to make sure that you speak "on your air" so that your voice is supported and you will be heard.

Another possible performance venue might be a rehearsal room or a large open room of some kind. Don't take anything for granted. Test the acoustics to get a sense of how your voice works within that space. Also get a sense of what it's like to make entrances and exits in this setting. Again, you'll probably see the audience, so become used to that and not afraid of it. It's part of this kind of performance.

Other kinds of theaters you may work in include small black box theaters, medium-size traditional theaters, and very large theaters. They all have things you need to adjust to. A black box theater might have similarities to a large room. A medium-size theater allows you to let your body and energy be a bit bigger. You never want to force your voice to be heard or move your body unnaturally. But you can allow your performance to be a little bit "extra" while still remaining truthful to the character.

It can be slightly intimidating to work in a large theater if you're not used to it. You are quite aware of the vastness of the stage and the black hole where lots of people may or may not be sitting. Don't become overwhelmed by the space, but embrace it. Spend as much time getting used to the stage as possible. And remember your character's wants and needs. What is the character *doing* in the play? What are the *actions*? This will help you let the physical space be part of your character's world.

Your Schedule

Maybe it seems silly to bring up scheduling when talking about artistic endeavors. But when a performer's time management gets out of balance, stress can easily slip in and get in the way of the artistic process. Besides, it can be surprisingly complex to balance activities such as going to class, rehearsing, and performing. In addition, you need to schedule time for everyday activities such as going to the gym, sleeping, doing homework, and eating. Many young actors find this quite challenging. I do find that making a master schedule—whether on your phone, in your journal, or on a large piece of paper that you hang on the wall—will really help. Some people use different colors for each activity. There is no one correct way to do it, but there will probably be a way that is most effective for you. There are also a number of useful articles and blog posts on time management for artists and creatives.

One way of mapping out your week is to put the essentials on your calendar first.

- Homework
- Classes
- Rehearsals
- Performances

Now add in important personal activities.

- Meals
- Exercise
- Sleep

Some things are easy to forget, but you need to make time for them as well.

- Laundry
- Commuting

This last item on the list is especially important. Shoot for being fifteen minutes early to rehearsals. You can use the time to warm up. And the last thing you want to do is rush to a performance and have to go straight on without preparing.

Acting Fundamentals

Somehow many performers feel that once they land a role they have to do something superhuman in order to justify their being cast—that it's necessary to knock it out of the park or nail it immediately. This is one way of looking at performances, but I have a different point of view that comes from my work with the Alexander Technique. For me, it's all about the process rather than an idealized vision of a big result. The latter can easily lead to tension and pushing.

Sometimes young actors tend to look outside themselves for inspiration. *The irony is that the keys to a good performance are already inside you.* It's sometimes hard to trust that you already have all you need. But that's where the Alexander principles can be helpful. If you focus on the individual tasks at hand, you will organically achieve a full, embodied performance.

Following are some examples of paying attention to the process versus the results:

- Notice what's happening for you physically on the way to the theater before a performance. What do you sense in your body? Are you noticing any points of tension?

- What's going on with your breathing as you head to the theater? Is the breath shallow or held? Or is it low and flowing?

- As you travel, think through your Alexander directions and the ideas of inhibition and direction.

- Be mindful of yourself as you walk up to the door and enter. Do you hold your breath, even in excitement?

- As you walk down the hall toward the green room, office, or dressing room, take time to look people in the eye and greet them. You can view this as a kind of warm-up.

Warm-Ups and Cool-Downs

Warm-ups can be practiced at home, at the theater itself, and even on your way to the theater (see page 123 for suggestions). Some warm-ups involve breath exercises and humming. You can also move the head gently from side to side and up and down to free the head on top of the neck. You can circle your shoulders gently as you walk. All these will help bring you more into your body.

Some people aren't clear why warm-ups are necessary. But think about cats and dogs. After they've had a night's sleep, or even a nap, they stretch their legs, backs, and whole bodies before they get on with their next activity. We can follow their example. When you warm up, you're all ready to go from your first entrance in the play. You then won't need to warm up on the stage, in front of the audience.

Just as it pays to spend a few minutes warming up, it's just as important to focus for a short period on cooling down after a performance. After all, you've just expended an extraordinary amount of energy on the stage or on the set. It's normal for you to be on a bit of a high because the stakes in many plays and films are very high. Your body will be full of adrenaline. Taking a few minutes to go through the Constructive Rest exercise (page 22), the Whispered "Ah" exercise (page 44), or the cool-down later in this chapter will help the adrenaline dissipate in a positive manner. Your breathing and body will return to an open, receptive state. Then you can carry on constructively with the rest of your night. You won't be locked into those imaginary circumstances. You can come back to your own reality. You want to leave the world of the play in the theater and leave the world of the film on the set at the end of each day.

Transformation

Transformation is the reason many actors want to become actors: the magic of becoming someone else. Sometimes the transformation can be subtle, barely discernible. Sometimes the transformation can be radical— we barely recognize the actor within the character. At its best, the transformation happens on several levels at once: physical, respiratory, vocal, kinesthetic, behavioral, emotional, and even spiritual, if you'd like to use that word. Somehow the actor uses the raw material of the self to create a whole other person. In some cases this will also involve help from costumes and makeup or a significant decrease or increase in weight. In other cases, like that of Peggy Ashcroft's Juliet, the transformation happens wholly from the inside. There is something rather magical about this process that the audience can sense and feel.

Transformation begins with the actor's choices about who and what the character is. Depending on your preference, and the piece you are working on, the transformation can initiate from the "inside" or "outside." Or you can work from both simultaneously. But however you work, ideally it begins with your understanding of the role and how it fits into the story of the play or film. It comes from an almost childlike belief in your ability to be someone else. In a sense, you want to embrace that belief, which will allow you to give yourself over fully to becoming the character.

JOURNAL

1   Write down what you like best and what you find most challenging about performing. What do you feel you'd like to address in your performing over the next few months?

2   Sketch out a routine that you feel would serve you best on the day of a performance. How will this affect your sleeping and eating routines? What would be ideal in your exercise schedule and in your warm-up for the performance?

3   Write down three goals for your performances over the next few months. For example, you might list, "Work on staying in the moment, connecting as deeply as possible with my scene partners, and remembering my physical freedom when performing."

Exercises

WARM-UP

• Stand with your back against the wall and your feet a few inches away from the wall. Your head is not against the wall. (It would be going back and down if it were.)
• Sense the support from the back of the wall.
• Think through your Alexander directions.
• Whisper "ah" three times (page 44).
• Think up as you bend your knees forward and slide down the wall a bit.

- Allow your lower back to let go.
- Straighten your legs and come back up to standing.
- Repeat two more times.
- Come away from the wall. Let your head lead up, and your body follow. Your core is gently engaged. Sense the support through your back as you walk around the room.
- Imagine you still have the support from the wall. Whisper "ah" a few more times.

This exercise allows you to use the support of the wall almost the way you use the support of the floor during Constructive Rest (page 22). Sliding down the wall allows the back to ease and lengthen, especially through its lower and middle regions. Your body will remember the sensation of lengthening as you come away from the wall and walk.

COOL-DOWN

- Sit quietly in a chair.
- Think through your Alexander directions.
- Let yourself sigh a few times.
- Sense your back against the back of your chair. Your seat against the seat of the chair. Your feet against the floor.
- Imagine your character slowly leaving your body. Sigh again.
- Allow your head to come down toward your chest. Let the weight of your head draw your spine toward the floor.
- Hang over, with your head between your legs. Sigh again.
- Roll yourself slowly up, building yourself up vertebra by vertebra. Your head comes up last.
- Imagine the last vestiges of your character leaving your body.
- Return to yourself and the rest of your day or evening.

Allowing yourself to be quiet after all of the energy expended in a show is a good idea. This exercise only takes a few minutes but will help calm the muscular and nervous systems. And it gives you the chance to consciously let go of the character. This is especially important when playing a character who is very intense.

PLAYING A CHARACTER WITH GOOD USE

- Stand with your feet a bit apart.
- Think through your Alexander directions.
- Be aware of being at your full height.
- Be aware of yourself in three dimensions: the front, back, and sides of your body.
- Sense yourself in the space—the floor beneath your feet and the space all around you, including above your head.
- Walk around the room, continuing to be aware of your full height and your three dimensions as you move.

Some characters are graceful and move well. This is an exercise that allows you to explore that. It's not a case of having "good posture." That's too static and held. Rather, this exercise is a way of exploring fluidity and elasticity in movement.

PLAYING A CHARACTER WITH IMPERFECT USE

- Stand with your feet a bit apart.
- Think through your Alexander directions.
- Be aware of being at your full height.
- Then imagine you are playing a character who slumps. Let yourself slump heavily down.
- Come back up to your full height.
- This time, rather than slumping heavily down, let your body take the shape of the letter c. Your spine stays lengthened within the curve.
- Walk around the room in this c shape.
- Return to yourself.

Of course not all characters use themselves well. Some of them might slump. But if you actually slump heavily down, this will tighten your throat and your rib cage, which will adversely affect the sound of your voice. Also, it will be hard on your back to slump for a two-hour performance. You can keep your torso long and wide and simply take on a slightly curved shape. It will look the same to the audience, but it will be much easier on you.

PLAYING A CHARACTER WITH A DIFFERENT BODY TYPE

- Stand easily.
- Be aware of your Alexander directions.
- Imagine the body type you want to portray.
- Allow that image to affect your body.
- Walk across the room, continuing to think of yourself as having that body type.
- Pause and come back to your own body type.
- Imagine the other body, let it affect you, and walk around the room maintaining that new way of being.

Some actors will make stereotypical choices when playing a character with a different body type. Rather than going for an end result and layering that on your body, try exploring what it would feel like to be someone else from the inside.

PLAYING A CHARACTER OF A DIFFERENT AGE

- Sit comfortably.
- Think through your Alexander directions.
- Think about the age that you want to play.
- Don't take on cliché characteristics of that age. Let the age affect you from the inside.
- Stand up and walk in a circle around the chair as that age.
- If it helps you, think of a specific person you know who is that age.
- Sit in the chair. How does your body feel different working with this imagery?

Sometimes student actors need to play either children or older people. Rather than jumping to a conclusion as to how a child or old person would move, take things slowly. Really imagine what it is like to be someone that age. What does that feel like inside your body? Heavier or lighter? Smooth or jerky? Let your impulses come from the inside rather than making an obvious physical choice.

PHYSICALITY AND SOCIAL STATUS

- Place a book or another object on the floor in the center of the room.
- Stand at one end of the room. Think through your Alexander directions.
- Think about the social status of your character—their background, upbringing, schooling, and the type of dwelling they live in.
- Allow those circumstances to affect your body from the inside.
- Walk across the room and pick up the book as the character. Return to the other end of the room.
- Then walk across the room and put the book down on the floor as yourself.
- Remember your character and their circumstances. Pick up the book as the character again. What are the differences between you and the character in terms of physicality?

Try seeing things from your character's point of view. Think about their background and how that would affect their body and movement. What kind of clothes would they wear? What would the fabrics feel like? Are they more athletic than you or less? Are they used to being treated or viewed in a certain way? Explore what this might be like.

PLAYING A CHARACTER YOU DON'T LIKE

- Choose a character you don't like.
- Don't think through your Alexander directions.
- Imagine being that character.

- Move about the room. Stand, sit, bend, and open the door. Turn the lights on and off.
- What did you notice about that character's movement? How was it similar to or different from your own?
- Now think through your Alexander directions. Let your breath be easy. Be as free as possible.
- Become the character again—from the inside. Repeat the activities you did before. Do you notice any differences after thinking through your directions?

Some of us have an aversion to certain types of roles. But it is part of the actor's job to be nonjudgmental. If you judge your character, the audience will sense it and will sense that you are commenting on the character rather than embodying them fully and authentically. When you give yourself over to understanding the character, you may find things about them to relate to.

WHEN YOU'RE FEELING ILL

- Sit down or lie down with a support under your head.
- Scan your body for tension.
- Think of easing your neck and shoulder muscles.
- Allow your back to melt.
- Let yourself be supported by the chair or the floor.
- Allow your breath to be even and deep.
- Place your hands at the bottom of your rib cage. This will remind you to keep your breathing low.
- Allow your whole body to soften from head to toe.

There are times when you need to perform even though you're not feeling your best. If you're very ill, you won't perform. But there are other times when you feel well enough to go on. You need to be kind to yourself. Give yourself extra time, and let your body and breathing be as easy as it can. Take things in stages.

DEALING WITH PERFORMANCE ANXIETY

At the first signs of performance anxiety (stage fright) or a panic attack, take the following steps:

- Become aware of your symptoms.
- Don't try to push the anxiety away: name it.
- Be in your body. Let it release as much as you can.
- Make sure you aren't holding your breath, making your breath shallow, or hyperventilating.
- Let yourself breathe slowly and easily: low and slow.
- Tell yourself, "I'm going to be okay. I'm ready. I'm prepared."

Stage fright or performance anxiety is something that happens for almost every performer at some point. Know that you are not alone. It's best to face the issue head on. Don't ignore it, or pretend it's not happening. The medical research on performance anxiety shows that the mind tends to race, the muscles tense, and breathing either gets held or some people hyperventilate. The research shows the best thing you can do is get the breath low and slow, and release the body as much as you can. This will help you quiet your mind and your fears. The Alexander Technique can be of invaluable help in this situation. The mantras listed above will also help with quieting fears. If you are working with an Alexander teacher, make sure to mention to them whether you are experiencing anxiety. Also, if stage fright is a persistent issue for you, a qualified therapist can work with you for a limited amount of time. Working with possible underlying psychological issues can really help.

THE COLOR EXERCISE

- Stand comfortably with your feet apart.
- Think through your Alexander directions.
- Imagine that your body is hollow.
- Choose a favorite color. Imagine the color swirling around inside your body.
- Walk around the room.

- Imagine that you leave footprints of the color on the floor. Imagine that the top of your head leaves a trail of color across the ceiling.
- Move your hands and arms. Imagine that your fingers leave a trail of color in the air wherever you move them.

This exercise is excellent for developing poise and stage presence. It gives you a look of self-possession and gracefulness. Focusing on the color inside and outside your body helps any self-consciousness evaporate. The exercise can also help to give you a sense of the *volume* of yourself, a sense of what's going on inside of you, not just on the surface.

Primary Exercise

TRANSFORMATION

- Stand in the center of the room.
- Close your eyes for a moment.
- Imagine a character you'd like to play.
- How tall are they? Are they your body type? What age? Where did they grow up?
- Open your eyes.
- Allow yourself to breathe in their rhythm.
- What is the character's "vibe?" Smooth or jerky? Fast or slow? Intense or calm?
- Let your body begin to take that on—from the inside.
- Allow the character to inhabit your body.
- Now walk. How does the character move differently from you? Experiment. But don't "put it on"—let it emerge.
- Let the transformation go. Come back to yourself.
- Allow your breath to flow and your body to be easy.
- Let yourself go back to the character and move as them again. Practice going back and forth between your physicality and theirs.

This is one of the primary exercises I use in teaching transformation. Walking is such a fundamental movement for every person who is physically able to do it. That's why it's one of the best places to begin *as you allow yourself and the character to merge.* Also, you can train yourself to come into and out of the character at will. The more you explore, the easier it will become. As Meryl Streep has said, empathy is at the heart of the actor's art. And as I see it, one of the best ways to build empathy for another person is to practice walking in their shoes.

CONCLUSION

Certain things catch your eye, but pursue only those that capture the heart.

NATIVE AMERICAN PROVERB

Be real. Be yourself.

And yet—be somebody else.

These are two of the most common and somewhat contradictory messages given to actors. Experts tell you to be authentically yourself—but be the character at the same time. You are meant to transform your body, voice, movement, thoughts, and feelings, then use these altered components to help create another human being in a play or film.

The trouble is, the experts don't always tell you how to do it. *How* are you supposed to be authentically yourself?

Another common piece of advice given to actors is "Relax." This is probably not what people really mean when giving this suggestion. Technically, the only way you can completely relax is to lie down so you have complete support throughout your whole body. This is not practical when performing a play.

So what do teachers and directors mean when they give suggestions like these?

The truth is, *they are probably seeing something that is getting in your way.* What they are most likely seeing is mental-physical tension and restriction. They know that if you get rid of these things, you will probably be more comfortable and more able to freely commit yourself to living truthfully under imaginary circumstances.

This book has offered suggestions on how to transform yourself—not by *doing* something but by *undoing.* The undoing, or untangling of tension from your mental, muscular, and nervous systems, is not as complex as it first may seem. It comes down to one of the simplest and shortest words in our language: no. You say no to tightness, restriction, holding, freezing, squeezing, pulling down and pulling in, forcing, and pushing. You say no to tension. You say yes to allowing, freeing, and letting go.

If it's so simple, why hasn't it everyone done it by now? Because the force of habit is very strong. The Alexander Technique process of awareness, inhibition, and direction is extremely effective. But it needs to be practiced over a period of time before it can change ingrown, habitual behaviors.

An important benefit of practicing the Alexander Technique is that those who do so tend to become more centered—that is, less rushed and more mentally-physically coordinated and balanced. If you choose, you can apply this broadly throughout your life to help you prioritize what is most important to you. F. M. Alexander called this **constructive consciou control**. A more contemporary phrase might be *constructive self-management*. It means maintaining your mental and physical poise as you go about your daily activities. If you feel yourself tightening and restricting, you practice the Alexander principles to bring yourself back on course.

In the beginning, you can use this book to help you—along with, ideally, the support of a certified teacher of the Alexander Technique in group or private lessons. But ultimately, you will become your own best teacher, because you are with yourself all the time. You will become aware of when you are going back into your old unconstructive habits, and you can guide yourself into an improved use of yourself. Eventually, you will approach your own development with an attitude of self-acceptance and a lack of self-judgment. You have the gift of conscious choice, which grants you the ability to grow, change, and see things in a new light.

The Alexander Technique literally helps you feel more "in your body." It improves your proprioceptive sense and increases your sensory awareness. We're so often thrown into situations that are new, unknown, and confusing. The world is ever changing, and the pace of that change is increasing. Learning how to use yourself with poise and grace will help you exercise your privilege of choice. You don't know what's going to happen next, but with an increased presence of mind–body, you are free to choose how you react.

The business professor Leon Megginson wrote, paraphrasing Charles Darwin, "It is not the most intellectual of the species that survives; it is not the strongest that survives; but *the species that survives is the one that is able best to adapt and adjust to the changing environment in which it finds itself"* (I added the emphasis).

Some of you know that you are bound for a career as a professional actor. Others of you are exploring the possibility of directing, screenwriting, or another career in theater or film. Still others may end up entering different fields. Whichever road you take, I suspect that you will look back at this time of studying acting as something special and unique. You are taking the time to explore the world through drama, work in close partnership with actors, directors, and other theater artists, and learn a great deal about your inner experience. Acting opens horizons inside you. It's something most people never have the opportunity to explore. It will inform your experience for the rest of your life.

Actors often see the world differently from other people. Some are idealistic; some more worldly. But they all tend to see things through a creative and artistic lens. They sometimes notice things that others take for granted. Some want to strike out in new directions and create something special and exciting. They may not want to settle for the average and mundane.

Whoever you are at heart, whatever your point of view—it is *yours*. The world of theater and film supports that individuality. And the Alexander Technique supports your self-identity and expression. The Alexander Technique is the most practical way I know to help you become most fully yourself, by helping ease your tensions and anxieties and encouraging you to take up your full mental, physical, and spiritual space. In that way, you can be your most natural self. You have a voice, and it deserves to be heard. And the best way to produce your authentic voice is from your fully expanded and expansive body.

APPENDIX A: INTERPRETING THE SOUND CONTAINER EXERCISE

The purpose of the Sound Container exercise is to look at yourself from a different point of view—to see yourself laid out in two dimensions, on a piece of paper. Take note of what you colored in and what you didn't. You might single out your mouth, your tongue, your rib cage, and your diaphragm as being important parts of your body in creating sound. But many people might not color in the cheekbones and the forehead—yet ideally there is a lot of vibration in these areas when making sound. Even the top and the back of the head is fertile ground for vibration. If you leave out some parts that can potentially vibrate when speaking and singing, it's possible that those regions of your body are not being fully activated when you make sound.

Also, the way you draw vibrations emanating from your body is telling. You may have drawn the vibrations coming out from your body and forward into the environment. But it's important to keep in mind that the vibrations flow up toward the ceiling, out to either side, and even from your back toward the wall behind you. Sound travels in all directions, even if the focus is mainly toward the people you are speaking to.

APPENDIX B: LIST OF EXERCISES

Chapter 1: Your Body

Exercises Part 1

Alexander Directions
Releasing Your Neck
Head Poise
Lengthening and Widening Your Torso
Opening Your Shoulders Part 1
Opening Your Shoulders Part 2
Releasing Your Arms
Softening Through Your Hands
Letting Go of Your Legs
Freeing the Feet
Constructive Rest

Exercises Part 2

Let Go of Your Body
Get Out of Your Head
Be Centered
Get Energized
Find Your Confidence
Primary Exercise: Presence

Chapter 2: Breathing

Freeing the Throat Part 1
Freeing the Throat Part 2
Breath Awareness
Releasing Your Breath

How Nerves Affect Your Breath
Finding Your Quiet, Open Breath
Learning About Your Breathing Habits
Observing Babies and Animals
Observing Great Actors
Hissing
Blowing Out Air
Humming
Primary Exercise: Whispered "Ah"

Chapter 3: Your Voice

Releasing the Larynx
Freeing the Base of the Tongue
Letting Go of the Jaw Part 1
Letting Go of the Jaw Part 2
Softening the Muscles at the Base of the Skull
Easing the Upper Face and Head
Opening through Your Chest
Releasing through Your Rib Cage
Physical and Vocal Vibration
Body into Sound
Telling a Story
Using Your Voice With an Open Body
Primary Exercise: Vibration throughout Your Whole Body

Chapter 4: Your Movement

Walking
Sitting
Sitting Efficiently
Sitting at the Computer
Bending
Lunging
How to Text
Using Stairs
Raising Both Arms
Looking Up and Down
Carrying Bags
Apparent Stillness

APPENDIX C:
LIST OF VIDEOS

To view a particular video, please visit its URL below or go to https://vimeo.com/channels/1488540.

Presence: https://vimeo.com/352648497
Whispered "Ah": https://vimeo.com/352648345
Vibration Through Your Whole Body: https://vimeo.com/352648244
Your Character's Movement: https://vimeo.com/352648099
Working with Resistance, Not Against It: https://vimeo.com/352647930
Aligning the Mind and Body: https://vimeo.com/352647346
Private Warm-Up: https://vimeo.com/352646769
Transformation: https://vimeo.com/352648587

GLOSSARY

acting from the inside out: In this tradition, the internal life and the "truth of the character" are seen as primary, whereas the externals will reveal themselves naturally.

acting from the outside in: A centuries-old tradition of working from external characteristics first. This includes what the character looks like, what they wear, what their movement is like, what dialect they speak, and, in certain forms of classical theater, what type they represent. From these externals one can begin to form the character's inner life.

active sitting: Maintaining optimal use of the self as you sit by releasing up into length and out into width and allowing your breath to flow.

Alexander directions: A specific type of intention, thinking, and mental cuing: "Let the neck be free, to let the head release forward and up, to let the torso lengthen and widen, to let the arms and legs release away from the body."

Alexander Technique: A method of education through which you learn how to recognize your unconstructive mind–body habits, consciously prevent them, and develop more positive and efficient ways of functioning by mentally cuing yourself.

apparent stillness: Appearing to be still without holding or freezing yourself in place; a pause or a suspension—letting go of unnecessary movement.

authentic voice: A voice that comes from your open physical instrument powered by free-flowing breath; a sound that vibrates healthfully, with natural overtones and undertones.

balance: An efficient equilibrium achieved in the absence of anything extraneous.

consciousness: A set of ideas, attitudes, and beliefs.

coordination: Managing the various parts of your body in a smooth and efficient manner so they work as a harmonious whole.

constructive conscious control: F. M. Alexander's term for a positive mental influence over the mind–body during daily activity.

correct mental attitude: F. M. Alexander's term for approaching things positively and with an open mind.

diaphragm: The primary muscle of breathing. It descends and ascends during respiration.

direction: Gentle guidance you give yourself in the moment after you become aware of a particular habit and decide you don't want to keep doing it anymore.

emotions: A strong feeling deriving from one's circumstances, mood, or relationships with others.

end-gaining: F. M. Alexander's term for going after results while paying little or no attention to the process.

ergonomics: An applied science concerned with designing and arranging things people use so that the people and things interact most efficiently and safely.

expanded field of awareness: Not restricting stimuli coming into your awareness but not being distracted by them, either.

fight-or-flight response: A stress reaction to a perceived threat. Several systems in the body respond in a strong way; also sometimes called the startle response.

flexibility: Using your body in a pliable and elastic way to allow for the freest possible range of movement, maximum lengthening, and healthful muscle tone.

focus: Consciously giving your attention to a task without undue mental or physical tightness and restriction.

gestalt: Something such as a structure or experience that, when considered as a whole, has qualities that are more than the total of all its parts.

habit: A behavior we repeat often, mostly without thinking about it.

head–neck relationship: The key to constructive central coordination, it involves balancing the head at the top of the spine.

inhibition: Saying no to an old habit, sometimes called a "positive no" or "withholding consent." You consciously decide you don't want to do something that is not the best for you.

intelligence: The ability to learn or understand or to deal with new or trying situations. *Also*: the skilled use of reason.

intercostal muscles: The muscles between the ribs. They are the secondary muscles of breathing. The ribs gently move out and in during respiration.

kinesthesia: The awareness of the position and movement of your body parts.

Method acting: The American interpretation of Stanislavsky's teachings. This often refers to Lee Strasberg's work as well as that of Stella Adler, Uta Hagen, Bobby Lewis, Michael Chekhov, Sanford Meisner, and other prominent acting teachers of the mid- and late twentieth century.

mind–body: An entity comprising the brain, the body, the mind, and behavior and including physical, emotional, mental, social, and spiritual elements.

mind-set: A series of ideas, concepts, and assumptions that influences the way you see yourself and the world.

momentum: The force that keeps an object moving or keeps an event developing after it has started.

monkey position: *See* position of mechanical advantage.

neuromuscular reeducation: Using your sensory awareness, your muscular system, and your nervous system to improve your balance, coordination, and movement.

onset: The moment right before you move or speak; *see also* vocal onset.

open, receptive state: A state of being at ease and coordinated in the mind, body, and breath, leaving you open to new experiences; similar to what some call "actor's neutral."

overbreathing: Forcing air in and out while breathing.

overconcentration: Hyperfocus on one thing to the exclusion of all else.

phonation: The process by which the movement of vocal folds and breath create sound.

poise: Not falling prey to old, unconstructive habits, either mental or physical.

position of mechanical advantage: Bending the knees and leaning forward from the hips without slouching from the waist or arching from the back.

postural tone: An appropriate amount of muscular effort in order to carry out an activity.

process oriented: Focusing on the means rather than the end; prioritizing the experience rather than the result.

psychophysical intelligence: Understanding—on an ongoing, developing basis—the ways in which mind and body work in unison to achieve the best possible functioning of the self.

psychophysical observation: Asking yourself what you are doing with your body, your mind, and your breathing and observing yourself almost as you would a stranger or a friend—nonjudgmentally.

pulling down: A physical collapse, or a forceful downward pull, through your torso.

redirecting: Renewing the thought of your Alexander directions in the midst of an activity.

resistance: Resistance to something such as a change or a new idea; a refusal to accept it.

respiration: The process of moving air into and out of the lungs, bringing oxygen into the body and expelling carbon dioxide.

sensory awareness: A sense of your inner and outer environment, helping create your understanding of your body in space, its positioning and movement, and the amount of effort it takes to create that movement.

sitting bones: Also known as the ischial tuberosity, these are two curved horseshoe-shaped bones at the base of the pelvis. They help you remain balanced as you sit.

Socratic question: A question or series of questions that stimulates students to come to their own conclusions by examining their thoughts and thinking processes.

somatizing: Manifesting unprocessed and sometimes unconscious fear, anxiety, stress, and mental and emotional tension in the body; physicalizing unexamined mental and emotional problems.

Stanislavsky, Konstantin: A legendary Russian theater practitioner, teacher, and author of books on acting theory and training. Born into a privileged family, Stanislavsky performed and directed as an amateur into early adulthood. He then cofounded the Moscow Art Theater with Vladimir Nemirovich-Danchenko. He was able to improve his own movement and coordination through awareness and practice. After studying with well-known teachers of voice, movement, and acting, he developed his own theories of actor training that became world famous. He also influenced many acting teachers who came after him, including Lee Strasberg, Sanford Meisner, Stella Adler, and many others.

startle response: *See* fight-or-flight response.

staying with yourself: Not losing yourself in what you are doing. Staying mentally and physically balanced as you engage in activity; being aware of yourself and your environment at the same time.

strength: Finding power and potency, vigor and vitality, in your self while maintaining these states over a period of time.

suboccipital muscles: The muscles at the base of the skull; the postural muscles that aid in the movement of the head.

tension habits: Tension that gets ingrained in the body. The most habitual movements and activities, such as walking, sitting, and standing, often have the strongest tension habits associated with them.

tension: Excess effort; more effort than is needed to accomplish an action.

tidal breathing: Breathing quietly when you're not engaged in a vigorous activity.

TMJ: Temporomandibular joint pain; can result in lockjaw, toothache, and difficulty chewing.

use of the self: The way you use yourself or function in your daily life mentally, physically, and emotionally.

vocal onset: The moment you begin to phonate.

willpower: The ability to control your own thoughts and behavior, especially in difficult situations.

BIBLIOGRAPHY

Allen, Glenn Seven. *The Singer Acts, the Actor Sings: A Practical Workbook for Living Through Song, Vocally and Dramatically*. London: Methuen Drama, 2019.

Bloch, Michael. *FM: The Life of Frederick Matthias Alexander*. London: Little, Brown, 2004.

Carrington, Walter. *Thinking Aloud: Talks on Teaching the Alexander Technique*. Berkeley, CA: Mornum Time Press, 1994.

Connington, Bill. *Physical Expression on Stage and Screen: Using the Alexander Technique to Create Unforgettable Performances*. London: Methuen Drama, 2014.

Gelb, J. Michael. *Body Learning: An Introduction to the Alexander Technique*. 2nd ed. New York: Henry Holt, 1994.

Hagen, Uta, and David Hyde Pierce. *Respect for Acting*. Hoboken, NJ: Jon Wiley & Sons, Inc, 1973.

Hanh, Thich Nhat. *How to Sit*. Berkeley, CA: Parallax Press, 2014.

Hanh, Thich Nhat. *How to Relax*. Berkeley, CA: Parallax Press, 2015a.

Hanh, Thich Nhat. *How to Walk*. Berkeley, CA: Parallax Press, 2015b.

Herrigel, Eugen. *Zen in the Art of Archery*. New York: Pantheon, 1953.

Huxley, Aldous. *Ends and Means: An Inquiry into the Nature of Ideals*. New York: Harper & Brothers, 1937.

Kapit, Wynn, and Lawrence M. Elson. *The Anatomy Coloring Book*. 4th ed. San Francisco, CA: Pearson, 2013.

National Center for Complementary and Alternative Medicine. "Mind–body Medicine Practices in Complementary and Alternative Medicine." National Institutes of Health: https://report.nih.gov/NIHfactsheets/ViewFactSheet.aspx?csid=102.

Sher, Barbara. *Live the Life You Love in Ten Easy Step-by-Step Lessons*. New York: Delacorte Press, 1996.

Stanislavsky, Konstantin. *Building a Character*. New York: Theatre Arts Books, 1949.

Stanislavsky, Konstantin. *My Life in Art*. Translated by Jean Benedetti. Abingdon, UK: Routledge, 2008.

Wolf, Jessica. *The Art of Breathing*. www.jessicawolfartofbreathing.com/.

Other Resources

Free visual anatomy app:
Visual Anatomy Lite by Education Mobile, www.edumobapp.com/product.html.

To find an Alexander teacher near you:
In America, American Society for the Alexander Technique:
http://amsatonline.org.
In the United Kingdom and Europe:
http://alexandertechnique.co.uk.

To invite Bill Connington to teach seminars, workshops, or classes, or to invite him to visit your college or school, please contact him at: billconnington@gmail.com.